CLINICAL PET

Developments in Nuclear Medicine

VOLUME 28

Series Editor: Peter H. Cox

The titles published in this series are listed at the end of this volume.

Clinical PET

edited by

R. BARES

Department of Nuclear Medicine,
Eberhard-Karls-University, Tuebingen, Germany

and

G. LUCIGNANI

INB-CNR, Department of Nuclear Medicine,
University of Milan, Scientific Institute H.S.,
Raffaele, Milan, Italy

KLUWER ACADEMIC PUBLISHERS

DORDRECHT / BOSTON / LONDON

Library of Congress Cataloging-in-Publication Data

Clinical PET / edited by R. Bares and G. Lucignani.
p. cm. -- (Developments in nuclear medicine ; v. 28)
Based on precongress meeting held in Dusseldorf, Germany prior to the 1994 Annual Meeting of the European Association of Nuclear Medicine.
Includes index.
ISBN-13:978-94-010-6624-2 e-ISBN-13:978-94-009-0309-8
DOI:10.1007/978-94-009-0309-8

1. Tomography, Emission--Congresses. I. Bares, R. (Roland) II. Lucignani, G. (Giovanni) III. European Nuclear Medicine Congress (1994 : Dusseldorf, Germany) IV. Series.
[DNLM: 1. Tomography, Emission-Computed--congresses. W1 DE998KF v.28 1996 / WN 206 C641 1996]
RC78.7.T62C556 1996
616.07'575--dc20
DNLM/DLC
for Library of Congress 96-25021

ISBN-13:978-94-010-6624-2

Published by Kluwer Academic Publishers,
P.O. Box 17, 3300 AA Dordrecht, The Netherlands.

Kluwer Academic Publishers incorporates
the publishing programmes of
D. Reidel, Martinus Nijhoff, Dr W. Junk and MTP Press.

Sold and distributed in the U.S.A. and Canada
by Kluwer Academic Publishers,
101 Philip Drive, Norwell, MA 02061, U.S.A.

In all other countries, sold and distributed
by Kluwer Academic Publishers Group,
P.O. Box 322, 3300 AH Dordrecht, The Netherlands.

Printed on acid-free paper

TABLE OF CONTENTS

FOREWORD

The 1994 Convention of the European Association of Nuclear Medicine (EANM) in Düsseldorf, Germany (Aug. 20 - 24) was preceeded by five precongress meetings. One of these was headlined "Clinical PET" and was most sucessfully organized by Roland Bares, Aachen (G) and Giovanni Lucignani, Milano (I). As the congress president, I felt very happy that it clearly was aimed at the clinical benefit of PET methods and at employment of this most elegant method in three important fields of patients care, viz. cardiology, neurology and oncology. Organizers, chairmen and speakers belong to the upcoming generation of young but already highly qualified nuclear physicians and physicists in Europe and Japan. Experienced physicians, they may be addressed as critical PET-users, added their view of patients demands.

PET started in the late seventies by combining physicists, chemists, physicians and engineers to bring cyclotron, radiochemistry, PET scanner and mathematical modelling into function (PET center). In the eighties, PET was further developed in some few research centers, employed in man to answer questions of fundamental interest and concern. However, as a logic consequence of physiological research in normals, followed by pathophysiologically guided research in selected patients, such "clinical research" has to end up in serious and critical clinical employment. This has first been restricted to some rather special clinical constellations as in some brain diseases. The next step gave insight into the heart and into coronary artery disease. Subsequently, it was found that PET may be employed in two conditions, viz. in PET centers and in satellite PET stations (PET scanner located in large university departments of nuclear medicine in proximity to a PET center, supported from there with transportable radiopharmaceuticals) as well. PET studies became larger, more clinically and benefit oriented, as for instance in hibernating myocardium. Futhermore, now based on the body of knowledge of medical faculties, they were used to test and to elucidate fields of proved indication in patients. Thus, PET left its former ivory tower. During the last years, oncologic questions were addressed and most elegantly answered also by employing satellite PET.

Today we face three areas of significance for PET, viz. basic research, clinical research and clinical employment. For the latter, development of powerful workstations yielded to combine PET data with SPECT data sets and to merge such slices of function with morphologically oriented slices from MRI or CT. This is an unique advantage if PET is intergrated into an university hospital. Diagnostic impact, therapy monitoring and prognosis are the goals for PET studies in such clinical environment. As in all nuclear procedures, radiation protection and quality assurance have to be considered.

However, if a method becomes a clinical tool, it has to face critical evaluation by stake holders and interested parties. Results and costs have to be compared to other diagnostic modalities. Referring physicians, health economists and official bodies have to be convinced of its clinical power.

The present book summarizes the lectures, given at this well frequented precongress meeting, comprizing basic pathophysiology, clinical demands for PET and clinical results of PET procedures in patients, already confirmed and widely accepted. It further illuminates future clinical goals to be reached if the most significant strategy is kept in mind. i.e. PET acts as a tool for both, reseachers and physicians. I hope that this message is carried out through this publication.

Prof. Dr. U. Buell
EANM Congress President , 1994

PREFACE

During the past decade Positron Emission Tomography (PET) has turned from a highly sophisticated tool developed for basic research in neurology and cardiology into an advanced nuclear medicine imaging technique ready for routine use. Along with remarkable technical improvements an overwhelming number of PET studies has been published covering not only scientific but also relevant clinical problems. Due to this rapid development comprehensive information about the current status of "clinical" PET is missing. It is the aim of this book to provide a critical overview about relevant applications of PET for all those who are beginning to run a PET facility or are planning to do so. Furthermore the book is dedicated to interested clinicians who are willing to utilize the diagnostic potential of PET.

In this book the applications of PET in neurology, cardiology, and oncology are discussed in three sections. In each section, following an introduction reviewing the present clinical demands, special diagnostic problems and their possible solution by PET are addressed. Results of conventional scintigraphic techniques are mentioned, too, and compared with PET. In a fourth section technical aspects (e.g. instrumentation, software) are presented including statements of representatives of leading manufacturers in the field of PET; readers willing to learn about PET radiopharmaceuticals will find in another recent book of this series an extensive review.

Since all of the papers were presented during the meeting "Clinical PET" held in Düsseldorf prior to the 1994 annual meeting of the European Association of Nuclear Medicine, they reflect current knowledge and state of the art information about this most exciting new field of Nuclear Medicine. We hope the readers will enjoy the book and take maximum profit from it for their personal work and an optimized patient care.

Roland Bares and Giovanni Lucignani
Tübingen and Milano, April 1996

LIST OF CONTRIBUTORS

Roland B. Bares Department of Nuclear Medicine, Eberhard-Karls-University, Roentgenweg 13, D-72076 Tübingen, Germany

Udalrich Buell Department of Nuclear Medicine, Technical University, Pauwelstrasse 30, D-52057 Aachen, Germany

Maike De Wit Department of Oncology and Hematology, University Hospital Eppendorf, Martinistrasse 52, D-20246 Hamburg, Germany

Ulrich Feine Department of Nuclear Medicine, Eberhard-Karls-University, Roentgenweg 13, D-72076 Tübingen, Germany
Co-authors: Roland Lietzenmayer and Wolfgang Mueller-Schauenburg

Karl Herholz Max Planck-Institute for Neurological Research, Gleueler Str. 50, D-50931 Cologne, Germany

Andy Holley General Electrics Medical Systems, Coolidge House, 352 Buckingham Avenue, Slough, Berkshire SL1 4ER, U.K.

Kazuo Kubota Department of Nuclear Medicine & Radiology, Institute for Development, Aging and Cancer, Tohoku University, 4-1 Seiryomachi Aobaku, SENDAI, Miyagi 0980-77, Japan
Co-authors: Susumu Yamada, Masatoshi Ito, Kenji Yamada, Takehiko Fujiwara, Roko Kubota, Kiichi Ishiwata, Hiroshi Fukuda, Taiju Matsuzawa, Masao Tada and Tatsuo Ido

Giovanni Lucignani Department of Nuclear Medicine, University of Milan, H.S. Raffaele, Via Olgettina 60, I- 20132 Milan, Italy

Jacques A. Melin Laboratory for Positron Emission Tomography, University of Louvain Medical School, Chemin du Cyclotron 2, B-1348 Louvain La Neuve, Belgium
Co-authors: Jean-Louis Vanoverschelde, Bernhard Gerber, Christian Michel, William Wijns and Anne Bol

Stefan P. Mueller Department of Nuclear Medicine, University Hospital Essen, Hufelandstrasse 55, D-45147 Essen, Germany

Hartwig Newiger Siemens Medical Systems AG, Nuclear Medicine, P.O. Box 3250, D-91050 Erlangen, Germany

Bernard Sadzot Department of Neurology, Cyclotron Research Center, University of Liege Sart Tilman, B- 4000 Liège 1, Belgium
Co-authors: René M.C. Debets, Eric Salmon, Cornelius W.M. van Veelen, Guy Delfiore, Alexander C. van Huffelen and George Franck

Christiaan Schiepers Department of Nuclear Medicine, University Hospital Gasthuisberg, Herestraat 49, B-3000 Leuven, Belgium

Udo Sechtem Department of Internal Medicine III, University of Cologne, Joseph-Stelzmann-Strasse 9, D- 50924 Cologne, Germany
Co-authors: Christian A. Schneider, Eberhard Voth and Harald Schicha

Ludwig G. Strauss Department of Oncologic Diagnosis and Therapy, German Cancer Research Center, Im Neuenheimer Feld 280, D-69120 Heidelberg, Germany

Juergen vom Dahl Department of Internal Medicine I (Cardiology), Technical University of Aachen, Pauwelstrasse 30 , D-52057 Aachen, Germany

Cornelis Weiller Department of Neurology, University Hospital Essen, Hufelandstrasse 55, D-45122 Essen, Germany

Part One:
PET in Cardiology

1

PET IN CARDIOLOGY: CLINICAL BACKGROUND

Christian A. Schneider, Eberhard Voth, Harald Schicha, Udo Sechtem

Positron emitting compounds and positron emission tomography (PET) have opened new windows for the understanding of physiological and pathophysiological mechanisms of myocardial metabolism, receptor physiology and blood flow. This chapter focuses on two areas of clinical relevance where conventional diagnostic techniques may be misleading and a more accurate technique is clearly needed: the exact documentation of the severity of the coronary artery stenosis as a basis for therapeutic planning and the identification of viable myocardium in patients after myocardial infarction.

Underestimation Of CAD By Coronary Angiography

The overwhelming majority of physicians, especially invasive cardiologists, regard coronary angiography as the objective standard for measuring atherosclerosis within the coronary arteries. The recent introduction of coronary ultrasound, however, has reminded us of the fact that coronary angiography clearly underestimates the degree and

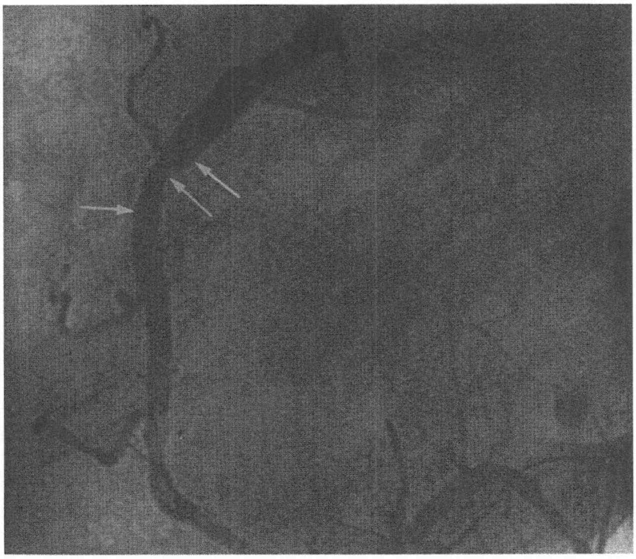

Figure 1a. Irregularities of the lumen of the right coronary artery throughout its course without angiographic evidence of high grade stenosis.

R. Bares and G. Lucignani (eds.) Clinical PET, 3–12.

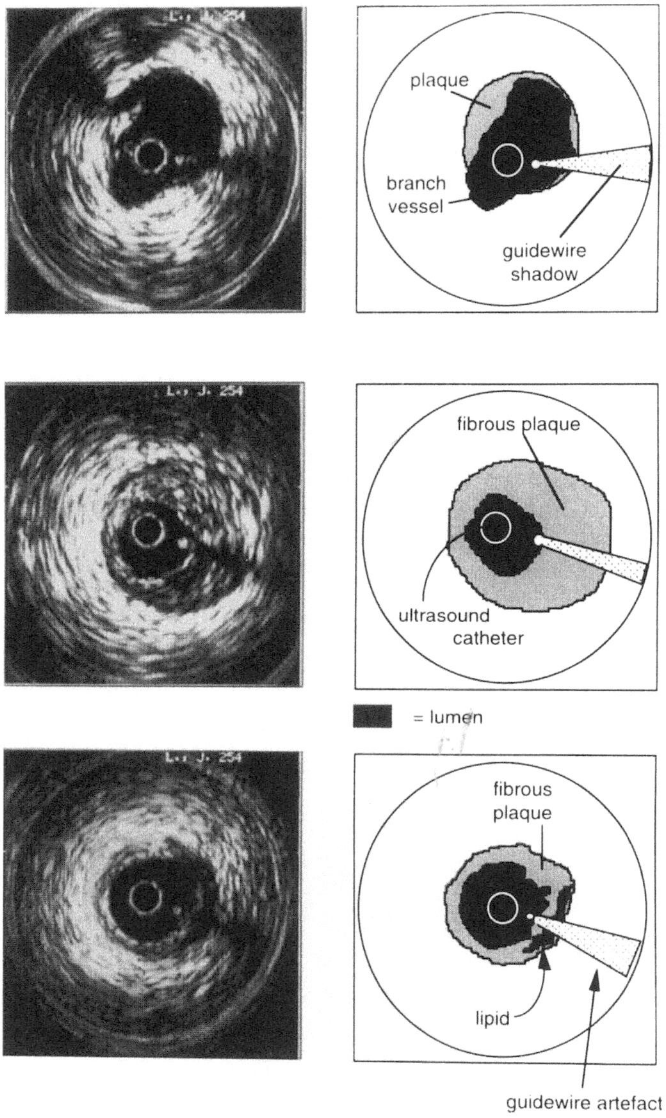

Figure 1b . Cross sectional ultrasound images at three levels of the right coronary artery indicated by the arrows in Fig 1a. Top: some plaque with calcification can be identified between 9:00 h and 12:00 h, the rest of the artery's circumference appears normal. Middle: luminal narrowing of more than 60% with a large fibrous plaque. The angiography does not detect this large plaque because the lumen is still fairly wide and the vessel has undergone remodeling to create space for the plaque. Bottom: concentric intimal thickening without a significant stenosis; the total vessel area is normal.

the extent of atherosclerotic disease. This observation has been repeatedly published by pathologists and cardiac surgeons but has not yet received much attention within the cardiology community. An example of the discrepant findings by angiography and intracoronary ultrasound is shown in Figure 1. Porter et al. [1] analysed 20 patients with angiographically proven CAD with stenosis <50% by quantitative angiography and intravascular ultrasound. Quantitation of the maximal narrowing of the coronary segments revealed a significantly more severe disease by ultrasound than the analysis of the same segment by quantitative angiography (36 (20%) vs. 19 (2%), p<0,001). In addition, 19 angiographically mildly diseased segements had a percent arterial area narrowing of >50% by ultrasound. Davies et al. [2] reported a case of a patient presenting with chest pain, angiography revealed normal coronary arteries except for an abnormality of the distal left mainstem coronary artery. Intravascular ultrasound revealed an extensive plaque in the distal left mainstem causing a 60% narrowing at one point. Because of this stenosis the patient underwent coronary bypass surgery and has been free of angina since the operation. Intracoronary ultrasound yields information about the extent of atherosclerosis [3], the composition and distribution of the plaque [4,5], the effects of angioplasty on the vessel [6,7] and the intimal changes after stent placement [8]. In addition, intravascular ultrasound can detect atherosclerosis in regions of focal vasospasm which seem to be normal on angiography [9].

Overestimation Of CAD By Coronary Angiography

In recent years intracoronary Doppler has transformed from a research tool to a diagnostic technique which can provide information about the results of coronary interventions [10], the effects of pharmacological interventions on coronary blood flow [11-13] and about stenosis severity [14, 15]. In a paper by Donohue et al. [16] 101 patients were examined by conventional coronary angiography and intracoronary Doppler wire. Angiographic data of stenosis severity were compared with translesional pressure gradients and translesional flow velocity. It could be shown that in angiographically intermediate stenosis (50-70%) the translesional pressure gradient varied between 0 and 85 mm Hg, making coronary angiography the least helpful method in determining the clinical significance of a lesion.

It is obvious that coronary angiography is not the ideal technique to determine the exact extent of coronary artery disease and not the best way of determining the immediate source of symptoms in patients with multi-vessel disease. In the age of PTCA for multi-vessel disease [17] it becomes increasingly important to identify whether a specific stenosis contributes to the symptoms. This is important because PTCA of the culprit lesion is often sufficient to abolish symptoms without catheter interventions at the other sites [18,19].

As shown above, conventional coronary angiography has shortcomings which limit considerably its use to answer clinically important questions: under- and overestimation of the stenosis severity occurs, the reproducibility of angiographic interpretation is poor [20,21] and the coronary angiogram lacks information about hemodynamic consequences of the disease. Finally, the angiogram is not even highly predictive of the site of a subsequent coronary occlusion [22, 23]. This lack of specific functional information about individual coronary stenoses makes it difficult to assess the physiological significance of an individual stenosis. In addition, dysfunction of the endothelium in patients with risk factors for coronary artery disease may precede structural changes of the coronary arteries and cannot be detected by conventional angiography [24].

The optimal tool to assess the morphological and functional extent of a stenosis in a single examination would be the combination of angiography, intracoronary ultrasound and Doppler echography. However, these techniques are expensive, increase the duration and the radiation burden of the examination and are not without risk for the patient. A single non-invasive test answering the important questions (identification of location and severity of a significant stenosis) in these patients would therefore be of considerable clinical importance. Conventional coronary angiography remains the "workhorse" of the invasive cardiologist: in most symptomatic patients it will provide the information needed for a correct therapeutic decision. However, with the introduction of newer scintigraphic techniques, including positron emission tomography (PET), the cardiologist has dependable tools to answer non-invasively and quantitatively the questions which remain unanswered by the angiogram.

Myocardial Viability

Since the introduction of the concept of "hibernating myocardium" by Rahimtoola in 1985 [25] one of the most common problems for the clinician caring for patients with coronary artery disease is to determine whether myocardium exhibiting a severe wall motion abnormality (akinesia or dyskinesia) is scarred or still viable. The correct answer to this question is not only important for the individual patient's choice of therapy (e.g.: medical, interventional or surgical therapy) but has tremendous clinical and economic impact because many patients are affected. For these reasons many different techniques have been used to distinguish viable from scarred myocardium such as echocardiography [26, 27] and scintigraphic techniques [28-30]. However, one has to keep in mind that the broad availability of these techniques may lead to some diagnostic overkill if they are employed in almost all patients with CAD and a history of myocardial infarction. Thus, the second part of this review will focus on two important clinical questions: 1. For which patient is the detection of viability important? 2. Can viability be reliably detected by conventional non-scintigraphic methods ?
Figure 2 shows the angiogram of a patient who had an episode of chest-pain four weeks before catheterization. Two weeks later an infarct was diagnosed in the ECG and several days later he had recurrent angina. The angiogram shows akinesia of the inferior wall. There are some irregularities of the circumflex artery, but the main lesion is the subtotal occlusion of the right coronary artery with incomplete opacification of the distal artery (Fig. 3, upper panel). After balloon angioplasty the right coronary artery fills promptly and completely (Fig. 3, lower panel). Was it justified to immediately proceed to angioplasty? In this patient a viability test was not warranted despite the akinesia of the inferior wall because viability was evident from the constellation of anginal symptoms, subtotal occlusion of the right coronary in the angiogram and the absence of significant lesions in other coronary arteries. The only possible reason for the patients continued symptoms was the lesion of the right coronary artery causing ischemia in the viable parts of the infarcted area in the inferior wall. A viability test after coronary angiogram would only have resulted in an expensive delay of the necessary therapeutic action.
Similar to patients with single vessel disease a viability study is not always necessary in patients with multi-vessel disease and reduced left ventricular function to make the correct therapeutic decision. Figure 4 shows the angiogram of a patient who had an inferior myocardial infarction in 1990 and developed severe angina 4 weeks before catheterization. The left ventricular angiogram shows regions of akinesia in the mid anterior wall, the apex and the apical portion of the diaphragmatic wall. The coronary

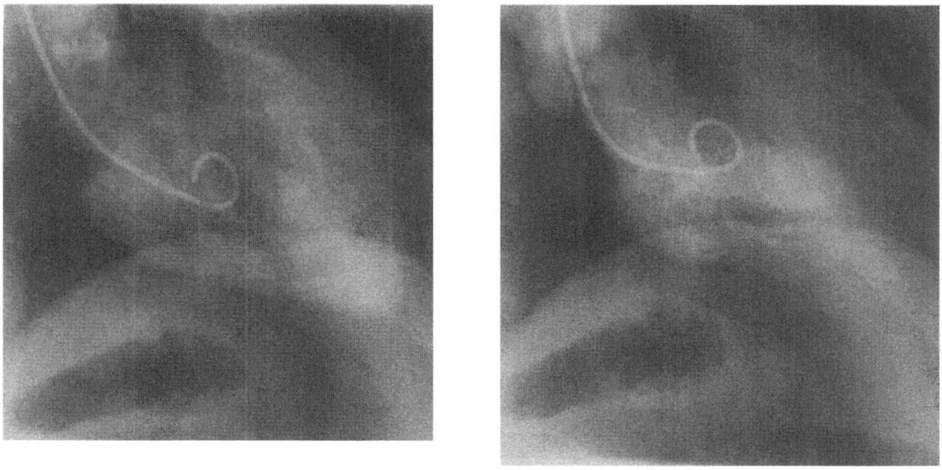

Figure 2. Angiogram of a 53 years old patient with inferior MI four weeks earlier, a pathological exercise stress test and recurrent angina during diastole (left panel) and systole (right panel).The angiogram shows normal contraction of the anterior and apical wall, whereas the diaphragmatic wall is akinetic.

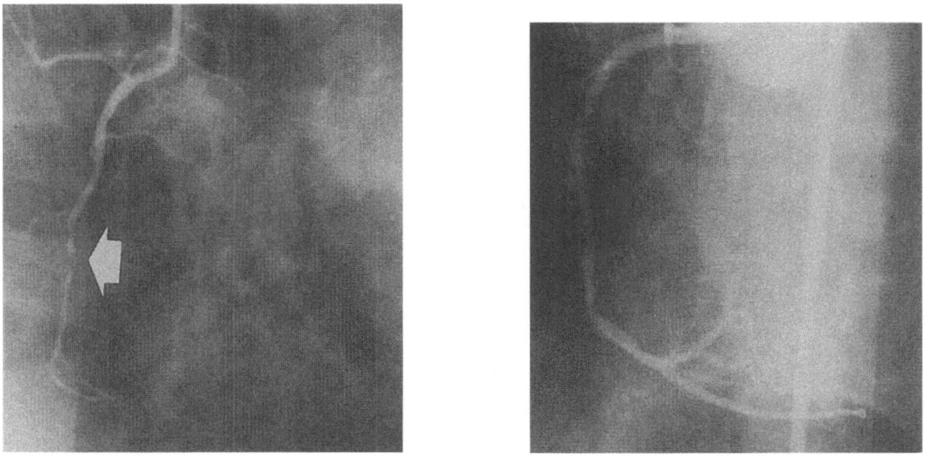

Figure 3. Coronary angiogram of the same patient exhibiting subtotal occlusion of the right coronary artery (left panel, large white arrow) and prompt filling of the right coronary artery after angioplasty (right panel).

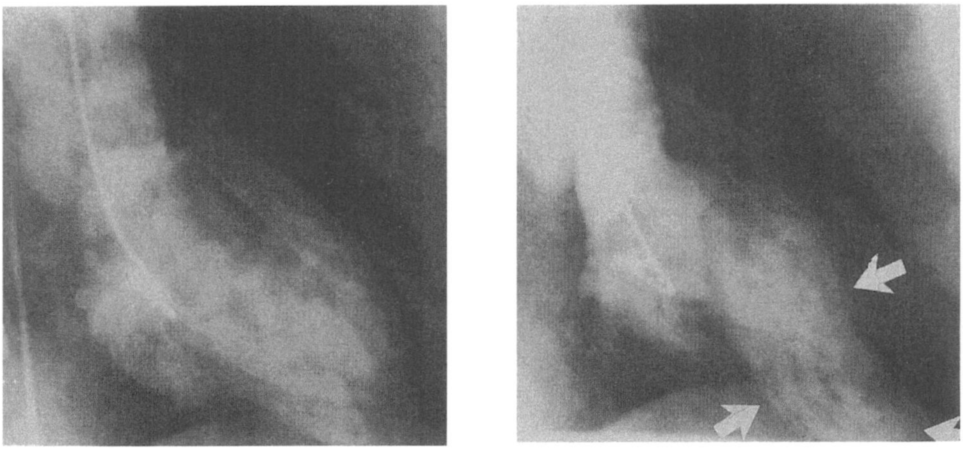

Figure 4 . Diastolic and systolic angiogram of a 59 years old patient with a history of inferior and anterior MI four years earlier, a pathological exrercise ECG and severe angina during daily life. The angiogram shows reduced left ventricular function with akinesia of the anterior wall, the apex and the diaphragmatic wall (small arrows).

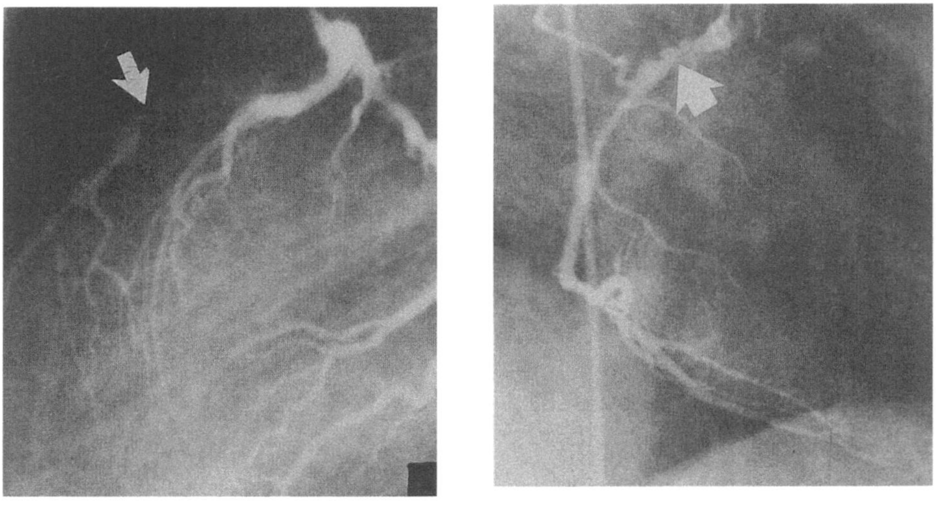

Figure 5. Coronary angiogram of the same patient as in figure 4 showing severe three vessel disease with subtotal occlusion of the left anterior descending artery (small white arrow) and a about 60% stenosis of the circumflex artery (left panel). The right coronary artery has a 80% proximal stenois (large white arrow, right panel).

arteries are severely diseased with high-grade lesions in the right coronary artery, a tight LAD stenosis and a moderate circumflex stenosis (Figure 5). This patient will profit from bypass-graft surgery irrespective of viability studies, because his left ventricular function is moderately reduced and he has severe three vessel disease [31]. All vessels should be bypassed because some viability in the area served by the left anterior descending artery is evident without viability studies due to the presence of contraction in the anterior wall near the apex.

Even in asymptomatic patients, information about myocardial viability can be derived from clinical and catheterization findings alone [32]: about 25% of regions with akinesia on the angiogram showed viability, defined as improved contraction after nitroglycerine in a second angiogram, despite the presence of Q-waves. Collateral filling of the infarct vessel is another important marker of viability: despite the presence of Q-waves, the presence of collaterals to the infarct vessel was associated with a 70% incidence of viability, whereas the absence indicated a low likelihood (67%) of viability [33,34]. Another way to estimate the presence of viability from the angiogram is the postextrasystolic improvement of contractility in the infarcted area. Popio et al. [34] showed that postextrasystolic potentiation in the infarcted area was a useful predictor of functional improvement after bypass surgery: of the seven patients with postoperatively increased ejection fraction, six (86%) had postextrasystolic potentiation in the preoperative ventriculogram compared to only 10/24 (42%) patients without such an improvement ($p<0,05$).

Thus, one can often make a reasonable judgement about viability from the improved contractility during the extrasystolic beat, the lesser degree of wall motion abnormality, the positive collateral status and of course simply from the presence of angina in a patient with single vessel disease. If one or more of these signs are present, viability studies will not add much information and may be superfluous.

The question of viability is much more difficult to answer in patients with severely depressed LV function, in whom a decision has to be made between medical, interventional, surgical and transplant therapy. In 1985, five year survival for patients with severely depressed left ventricular function (ejection fraction < 25%) was less than 30% for medical therapy and about 70% after coronary artery bypass surgery [35]. The poor prognosis for these patients with medical therapy has not changed with the advent of vasodilators [36]. It is currently unknown, whether the addition of low dose beta-blocking therapy will improve outcome. Luciani et al. [36] has recently reported on 143 patients with CAD and an ejection fraction of <30%. Patients received medical treatment, coronary bypass surgery or heart transplantation in a non-randomized fashion. The patients with bypass surgery or heart transplantation had a six year survival of about 80%, whereas the six year survival in patients on medical therapy was only 28%. The better survival of patients with bypass surgery can be partially explained as a consequence of the functional improvement of hibernating myocardium. However, in view of a perioperative mortality of about 10% for coronary artery bypass surgery in patients with low ejection fraction, is it not better to refer such a patient immediately for cardiac transplantation? The answer to this question depends largely on the amount of viable hibernating myocardium that will eventually recover its contractile function after revascularization. In patients with severely depressed left ventricular function ^{201}Tl and 2-[^{18}F]fluoro-2-deoxy-D-glucose ([^{18}F]FDG) and PET have been employed [36, 37] to identify viable myocardium and select patients for bypass surgery. Ragosta et al. [37] have shown in this patient population that a preoperative quantitative planar rest-redistribution ^{201}Tl scan reliably identified residual viability in akinetic regions. Over 70% of segments with normal or mildly reduced ^{201}Tl uptake had improved function after bypass surgery. Consequently, postoperative ejection fraction increased

significantly from 27% to 40% in patients with more than seven akinetic but viable segments. Similar data have been presented by Dreyfus et al. [38] who included an additional [^{18}F]FDG-PET scan in patients with negative ^{201}Tl scan. Only patients with a positive viability test underwent bypass surgery. After 6 to 10 months of follow-up the mean ejection fraction had increased significantly from 23% to 39%.
Thus, myocardial revascularization of patients with depressed left ventricular function and evidence of hibernation will improve global ejection fraction and survival and can thus be an alternative to transplantation.

Conclusions

Despite the availability of so many non-invasive and invasive techniques to diagnose CAD, more reliable, non-invasive quantitative methods for the detection and the assessment of the extent of CAD are still needed. There is a danger to overuse the excellent non-invasive techniques available today when viability after MI is the diagnostic question. Many therapeutic decisions can be made correctly on the basis of clinical and invasive information without viability studies. The patients in whom such viability studies are clearly warranted are those with extremly reduced left ventricular function in whom the therapeutic choice is between bypass grafting or transplantation. PET has the potential to be such a test but its ability to hold this promise when used as a clinical workhorse has yet to be demonstrated.

References

1. Porter TR, Sears T, Xie F et al. Intravascular ultrasound study of angiographically mildly diseased coronary arteries. J Am Coll Cardiol 1993; 22: 1858-65.
2. Davies SW, Winterton SJ, Rothmann MT. Intravascular ultrasound to assess left main stem coronary artery lesion. Br Heart J 1992; 68: 524-6.
3. Gerber TC, Erbel R, Görge G, Ge J, Rupprecht H-J, Meyer J. Extent of atherosclerosis and remodelling of the left main coronary artery determined by intravascular ultrasound. Am J Cardiol 1994; 73: 666-71.
4. Sheikh, KH, Harrison JK, Harding MB et al. Detection of angiographically silent coronary atherosclerosis by intracoronary ultrasonography. Am Heart J 1991; 121: 1803-07.
5. Nissen SE, Gurley JC, Grines CL et al. Intravascular ultrasound of lumen size and wall morphology in normal subjects and patients with coronary artery disease. Circulation 1991; 84: 1087-99.
6. Tobis JM, Mallery JA, Gessert J. Intravascular ultrasound cross-sectional arterial imaging before and after balloon angioplasty in vitro. Circulation 1989; 80: 873-82.
7. Honye J, Mahon DJ, Jain A et al. Morphological effects of coronary balloon angioplasty in vivo assessed by intravascular ultrasound imaging. Circulation 1992; 85: 1021-25.
8. Chokshi SK, Hogan J, Desai V et al. Intravascular ultrasound assessment of implanted endovascular stents (abstr). J Am Coll Cardiol 1990; 15: 29A.
9. Yamagishi M, Miyatake K, Tamai J, Nakatani S, Koyama J, Nissen SE. Intravascular ultrasound detection of atherosclerosis at the site of focal vasospasm in angiographically normal or minimally narrowed coronary segments. J Am Coll Cardiol 1994; 23: 352-57.

10. Bach RG, Kern MJ, Bell C, Donohue TJ, Aguirre F. Clinical application of coronary flow velocity for stent placement during coronary angioplasty. Am Heart J 1993; 125: 873-77.
11. Wilson RF, Wyche K, Christensen BV, Laxson DD. Effects of adenosine on human coronary arterial circulation. Circulation 1990; 82: 1595-1606.
12. Kern MJ, Deligonul U, Aguirre F, Hilton TC. Intravenous adenosine: Continous infusion and low dose bolus administration for determination of coronary vasodilator reserve in patients with and without coronary artery disease. J Am Coll Cardiol 1991; 18: 718-29.
13. Di Mario C, Strikwerda S, Gil R, de Feyter PL, de Jaegere P, Serruys PW. Response of conductance and resistance vessels to scalar concentrations of acetycholine: assessment with quantitative angiography and Doppler echography in 29 patients with coronary artery disease Am Heart J 1994; 127: 514-31.
14. Nakatami S, Yamagishi M, Tamai J, Takai H, Haze K, Miyatake K. Quantitative assessment of coronary artery stenosis by intravascular Doppler catheter technique. Circulation 1992; 85: 1786-1791.
15. Kenny A, Shapiro LM: Identification of coronary artery stenoses and poststenotic blood flow patterns using a miniture high frequency epicardial transducer: Circulation 1994; 89: 731-39.
16. Donohue TJ, Kern MJ, Aguirre FV et al. Assessing the hemodynamic significance of coronary artery stenoses: analysis of translesional pressure-flow velocity relations in patients. J Am Coll Cardiol 1993; 22: 449-58
17. Hamm CW, Reimers J, Ischinger T et al. A randomized study of coronary angioplasty compared with bypass surgery in patients with symptomatic multivessel coronary disease. N Engl J Med 1994: 331: 1037-43.
18. DeFeyter PJ, Serruys PW, Arnold A et al. Coronary angioplasty of the unstable angina related vessel in patients with multivessel disease. Eur Heart J 1986; 7:460-7
19. Wohlgelernter D, Cleman M, Highman HA, Zaret BL. Percutaneous transluminal coronary angiography of the Ñculprit lesionì for management of unstable angina pectoris in patients with multivessel coronary artery disease. Am J Cardiol 1986; 58: 460-4.
20. Shub C, Vliestra RE, Smith HC, Fulton RE, Elveback LR. The unpredictable progression of coronary artery disease: A serial clinical-angiographic analysis. Mayo Clin Proc, 1981; 56: 155-60
21. Zir LM, Miller SW, Dinsmore RE et al. Interobserver variability in coronary angiography. Circulation 1976: 53: 627-32.
22. Giroud D, Li JM, Urban P, Meier B, Rutishauser W. Relation of the site of acute myocardial infarction to the most severe coronary arterial stenosis at prior angiography. Am J Cardiol 1992; 69: 729-732.
23. Little WC, Constantinescu M, Applegate RJ et al. Can coronary angiography predict the site of subsequent myocardial infarction in patients with mild-to-moderate coronary artery disease? Circulation 1988; 78: 1157-66.
24. Reddy KG, Nair RN, Sheehan HM, Hodgson J McB. Evidence that selective endothelial dysfunction may occur in the absence of angiographic or ultrasound atherosclerosis in patients with risk factors for atherosclerosis. J Am Coll Cardiol 1994; 23,:833-43.
25. Rahimtoola S. The hibernating myocardium. Am Heart J 1989; 117:211-221.
26. Barilla F, Gheorghiade M, Kahja F, Goldstein S. Low-dose dobutamine in patients with acute myocardial infarction identifies viable but nor contractile myocardium and predicts the magnitude of improvement in wall motion abnormalities in response to coronary revascularization. Am Heart J 1991;122:1522-31.
27. Baer FM, Voth E, Deutsch HJ, Schneider CA, Schicha H, Sechtem U. Assessment of viable myocardium by dobutamine transesophageal echocardiography and comparison with Fluorine-18 Fluorodeoxglucose Positron Emission Tomography. J Am Coll Cardiol 1994; 24: 343-53.

28. Tamaki N, Ohtani H, Yonekura Y et al.Significance of fill-in after thallium-201 reinjection following delayed imaging: comparison with regional wall motion and angiographic findings. J Nucl Med 1990; 31: 1617-23
29. Dilzisian V, Freedman NMT, Bacharach SL, Perrone-Filardi P, Bonow R. Regional thallium uptake in irreversible defects. Circulation 1992; 85: 627-34.
30. Perrone-Filardi P, Bacharach SL, Dilsizian V, Maurea S, Frank JA, Bonow R. Regional left ventricular wall thickening. Relation to regional uptake of 18-Fluorodeoxyglucose and 201 Tl in patients with chronic coronary artery disease and left ventricular dysfunction. Circulation 1992; 86: 1125-37.
31. Rahimtoola SH. A perspective on the three large multicenter randomized clinical trials of coronary bypass surgery for chronic stable angina. Circulation 1985; 72(supplV)V123-35.
32. Banka VS, Bodenheimer BB, Helfant RH. Determinants of reversible asynergy. Effect of pathologic Q waves, coronary collaterals and anatomic location. Circulation 1974; 50: 714-19.
33. DiCarli M, Sherman T, Khanna S. Myocardial viability in asysnergic regions subtended by occluded coronary arteries: Relation to the status of collateral flow in patients with chronic artery disease. J Am Coll Cardiol 1994; 23: 860-68.
34. Popio KA, Gorlin R, Bechtel D, Levine JA. Postextrasystolic potentiation as a predictor of potential myocardial viability: preoperative analyses compared with studies after coronary bypass surgery. Am J Cardiol 1977; 39: 944-53.
35. Pigott JD, Kouchoukos NT, Oberman A, Cutter GR. Late results of surgical and medical therapy for patients with coronary artery disease and depressed left ventricular function. J Am Coll Cardiol 1985; 5: 1036-45.
36. Luciani GB, Faggian G, Razzolini, Livi U, Bortolotti U, Mazzucco A. Severe ischemic left ventricular failure: Coronary operation or heart transplantation? Ann Thorac Surg 1993; 55: 719-23.
37. Ragosta M, Beller GA, Watson DD, Kaul S, GimpleLW. Quantitative planar rest-redistribution 201Tl imaging in detection of myocardial viability and prediction of improvement in left ventricular function after coronary bypass surgery in patients with severely depressed left ventricular function. Circulation 1993; 87: 1630-41.
38. Dreyfus GD, Duboc D, Blasco A et al. Myocardial viability assessment in ischemic cardiomyopathy: benefits of coronary revascularization. Ann Thorac Surg 1994; 57:1402-08.

2

ASSESSMENT OF MYOCARDIAL PERFUSION BY PET

Jacques A. Melin, Jean-Louis Vanoverschelde, Bernhard Gerber, Christian Michel, William Wijns, Anne Bol

Several tracer approaches have been proposed for the assessment of myocardial perfusion with positron emission tomography (PET) in the clinical setting. These include nitrogen-13 (^{13}N) labelled ammonia, oxygen-15 (^{15}O) labelled water, rubidium-82 (^{82}Rb) and potassium-38 (^{38}K). These tracers require a local cyclotron for production, except for ^{82}Rb which may be delivered directly to the patient from an on-site generator.
There are two specific clinical applications of PET that have been proposed for the evaluation of patients with coronary artery disease (CAD) [1-3]. The first is the noninvasive detection of CAD and estimation of the severity of the disease. This is performed using a PET perfusion agent at rest and during pharmacologic vasodilation. A unique application of PET is the noninvasive calculation of absolute regional myocardial perfusion at rest and during vasodilation in humans using [^{15}O]water or [^{13}N]ammonia. However, most centers rely on the qualitative interpretation of ^{82}Rb or [^{13}N]ammonia images for the detection of CAD and the assessment of its severity. The second clinical application of PET is the assessment of myocardial viability in CAD patients with left ventricular dysfunction. The most common approach is to determine whether metabolic activity assessed by 2-[^{18}F]fluoro-2-deoxy-D-glucose ([^{18}F]FDG) is preserved in regions with reduced perfusion, thus indicating tissue viability.
In this chapter, we will review the clinical studies showing the evidence of a potential impact of qualitative and quantitative PET perfusion imaging for the diagnosis of CAD and for the assessment of its severity.

Diagnosis Of Coronary Artery Disease

Although single photon emission tomography (SPET) is used routinely in the clinical setting for this purpose, PET diagnostic accuracy for CAD has been investigated and compared with SPET. The anticipated improvement of diagnostic performance with PET is due to its superior spatial resolution resulting in increased sensitivity and to its ability to correct for attenuation, thus improving specificity.
Studies performed in about 500 patients who underwent rest and pharmacologic stress perfusion imaging using ^{82}Rb or [^{13}N]ammonia have reported sensitivities for CAD ranging from 87 to 97% and specificities ranging from 78 to 100% [4-8]. All these studies used qualitative or semi-quantitative PET protocols, including visual interpretation or circumferential profiles or polar maps types of analysis. Excellent PET

R. Bares and G. Lucignani (eds.) Clinical PET, 13–23.

image quality are indeed obtainable with ^{82}Rb and [^{13}N]ammonia with a high contrast between myocardial and underlying lung tissue or blood pool.

Only some of these studies directly compared PET and ^{201}Tl SPET in the same patient population. In a first study [6] performed in 51 patients studied by exercise ^{201}Tl SPET and dipyridamole [^{13}N]ammonia PET, the sensitivity of SPET (96%) and PET (98%) was similar. Specificity was not addressed because only 3 patients did not have CAD. In terms of identification of significant stenosis of individual coronary arteries, again the SPET data (81% sensitivity and 94% specificity) compared favorably with the PET data (88% sensitivity and 90% specificity). In a second study [7] involving 135 patients studied by dipyridamole-handgrip ^{201}Tl SPET and ^{82}Rb PET, the sensitivity was 93% for PET as compared to 76% for SPET and this was achieved with a similar specificity. In a third study [8] of 81 patients, similar sensitivities between ^{201}Tl SPET (using either exercise or dipyridamole) and ^{82}Rb PET (using dipyridamole-handgrip) were obtained for the diagnosis of CAD (90 and 87% respectively) and of individual coronary artery stenosis (65 and 64%). However, PET achieved higher specificity than SPET, both in the identification of CAD (82 and 57%, respectively) and in the detection of individual coronary artery stenosis (92 and 84% respectively). Lastly, a subset of 46 patients in a study by Demer et al. [5] had undergone both PET and SPET. This particular study showed that PET identified better than SPET those CAD patients with moderately severe (coronary flow reserve of <3) and with mild disease (flow reserve of 3-4).

Altogether, in the published series of patients with coronary angiography, there is a trend for a better sensitivity and specificity of qualitative or semi-quantitative PET as compared to SPET, both for the diagnosis of CAD and for the localization of individual stenosis. Using the published PET data in terms of diagnostic performance, Patterson et al [9] have compared cost-effectiveness of clinical algorithms to diagnose CAD with a comparison of exercise ECG, ^{201}Tl SPET, PET and coronary angiography. Their main conclusions were that the a priori probability of CAD should be considered when selecting a clinical algorithm and, doing so, stress PET was the more cost-effective test in patients with a probability of CAD <0.70 and angiography has the best cost-effectiveness in patients with a probability of CAD >0.70. More definitive comparative studies with comparable expertise in PET and SPET imaging should be performed in specific clinical subsets or situations in which SPET has been shown to lack diagnostic performance : obese patients, females, left bundle branch block, dilated cardiomyopathies, left ventricular hypertrophy. Also, sequential diagnostic strategies should be tested involving PET only in those patients with discordant results between exercise ECG and ^{201}Tl or with equivocal ^{201}Tl interpretation.

Assessment Of The Severity Of Coronary Artery Disease

Studies have been performed in the resting conditions and during pharmacologic vasodilation for the assessment of the severity of CAD. For this purpose, not only the intrinsic capabilities of PET perfusion imaging (spatial resolution and attenuation correction) are important but also the possibilities of quantifying myocardial perfusion in absolute terms, i.e. in ml/min/g. If PET measures the time course of both the arterial input function and the myocardial tissue concentration, absolute values of myocardial perfusion are obtainable by incorporating these quantities in a suitable physiologic model which takes into account the kinetics of the injected tracer. Experimental animal studies have shown the feasibility and accuracy of quantitative estimates of myocardial perfusion with [^{15}O]water [10-14], [^{13}N]ammonia [13-15] and ^{82}Rb [16].

RESTING STUDIES

After myocardial infarction, PET studies have demonstrated that revascularized infarcts have higher absolute flow values and are, therefore, more likely to contain a significant amount of viable tissue. Repeat measurements of myocardial blood flow with [^{15}O]water in 7 patients at day 1, 2 and 9 after early thrombolysis for acute myocardial infarction showed prompt restoration of nutritive perfusion in all but one patient [17]. Another study of myocardial blood flow using [^{13}N]ammonia was performed in 22 patients 86 ± 38 hours after acute myocardial infarction [18]. Ten out of the 22 patients were revascularized with either thrombolysis or PTCA. A wide range of myocardial blood flow values (from 0.1 to 0.9 ml/min/g) was measured in the infarcted regions. Flow in the infarcted segments that were shown to be metabolically active with [^{18}F]FDG imaging was higher (0.6 ± 0.2 ml/min/g) than in nonviable ones (0.3 ± 0.1 ml/min/g; $p < 0.05$). In another series of 15 patients with reperfused myocardial infarction that were studied 42 ± 25 days after the acute event, transmural flow averaged 0.8 ± 0.1 ml/min/g in remote segments, 0.7 ± 0.2 ml/min/g in adjacent, and 0.5 ± 0.1 ml/min/g in segments located in the center of the infarcted area [19]. Similar findings have been reported in 26 patients with chronic healed infarctions studied 44 ± 65 months after the event [20]. In this study, the presence of viable myocardium was very unlikely if basal myocardial blood flow was less than 0.25 ml/min/g. Using semi-quantitative estimates of ^{38}K myocardial uptake, Pierard et al. [21] already showed that a preserved myocardial perfusion is a good predictor of myocardial viability.

We have assessed the best predictors of postrevascularisation improvement of both regional and global left ventricular function in patients with sustained anterior wall dysfunction with and without a previous myocardial infarction [22, 23]. Among all absolute and relative PET variables investigated in this study, absolute myocardial blood flow was the most significant predictor for the return of left ventricular function after revascularization. Additional information was required only in patients with reduced absolute blood flow values. In these patients, assessment of regional glucose extraction appeared to be the most useful.

Lastly, resting PET absolute measurement of myocardial perfusion has allowed to gain some insights on the pathophysiology of left ventricular dysfunction in the absence of myocardial infarction or ongoing ischemia. We were able to demonstrate that myocardial stunning did indeed occur in human subjects and this was shown following attacks of unstable angina with persistent anterior wall dysfunction despite successful angioplasty of the culprit lesions. All these patients resumed normal regional function during the follow-up and at the time of the PET study, a few hours after the PTCA, they showed normal levels of myocardial perfusion and oxygen consumption despite abnormal regional function [24]. We have also investigated the mechanism of regional wall dysfunction in the so-called hibernating conditions as described by Rahimtoola [25]. We studied symptomatic patients with CAD, no previous myocardial infarction and complete chronic occlusion of a major coronary artery [26]. In these patients, the myocardium that was normally supplied by the occluded vessel had thus become totally dependent on the collateral flow. Some of these patients presented with a completely normal left ventricular function, while others displayed severe regional dysfunction despite no previous infarction. This latter group of patients fulfilled the criteria for chronic hibernation, as defined by Rahimtoola. We observed that despite a marked reduction in external work, dysfunctional collateral dependent myocardium remains metabolically active as demonstrated by the nearly normal basal flow and oxygen consumption and by the increase in [^{18}F]FDG uptake relative to flow (Table 1).

Table 1. Myocardial blood flow, exogenous glucose uptake, oxidative metabolism in remote and collateral-dependent myocardium

	rMBF	rMGU	FDG/NH_3	k
Patients with normal anterior wall motion				
Remote segments (n=25)	78±8[a]	33±12[a]	1.1±0.1	0.058±0.008[a]
Collateralized segments (n=18)	75±16[b]	33±11[a]	1.2±0.2	0.054±0.010[a]
Patients with anterior dysfunctional myocardium				
Remote segments (n=35)	92±23	42±20	1.3±0.6	0.068±0.020[c]
Collateralized segments (n=30)	68±17[b]	38±16	1.9±1.6[a]	0.049±0.015[c]

FDG/NH_3, ratio of $[^{18}F]$deoxyglucose to $[^{13}N]$ammonia relative uptake;
k (min^{-1}), slope of ^{11}C-acetate clearance;
rMBF: regionalmyocardial blood flow ($mL.min^{-1}.100g^{-1}$)
rMGU: regional myocardial glucose uptake ($\mu mol.min^{-1}.100\ g^{-1}$).
[a]$p<0.05$, [b]$p<0.01$, [c]$p<0.001$ vs remote segments of patients with dysfunction.
(From reference 26)

Thus, the data in this model do not support the hypothesis that chronic dysfunction results from a chronic reduction in resting flow. The contention that flow is decreased in "hibernating" states has been based on clinical studies on the relative distribution of flow tracers such as ^{201}Tl or ^{82}Rb. The interpretation of these scintigrams usually assumed that the segment with maximum tracer uptake have normal flow. However, perfusion scintigraphy only provided estimates of relative differences in tracer distribution. A seemingly decreased perfusion to a dysfunctional segment may well result from an absolute increase in flow to the remote hyperfunctioning tissue, as shown in this study by the quantitative measurement of transmural blood flow with $[^{13}N]$ammonia. From this study, a proposed working hypothesis for explaining chronic dysfunction, i.e. repeated episodes of ischemia and stunning, has to be further tested in patients and in experimental preparations mimicking the hibernating syndromes [27].

A methodological issue should be addressed at this stage since myocardial perfusion is often measured in the previously described conditions in dysfunctioning myocardial areas. In a dog model, artifactual reductions up to 36% decrease in apparent tracer concentration were caused by the reduced systolic thickening of areas made transiently ischemic [28]. This visual interpretation of uncorrected images could have lead to erroneous hypothesis regarding the severity of the flow deficits in "hibernating" myocardium. Clearly, visual flow defects in asynergic areas need to be shifted upwards in order to account for the offset imposed by the partial volume effect. The finite resolution effects are thus of major importance for quantification and one can attempt to correct for these effects if the actual geometric dimensions of the object and the resolution function of the scanner are known. A method consists of including finite resolution effects as additional parameters in the operational equation of the models. Bergmann et al. [11] estimated both correction factors (recovery and spillover) as additional fitted parameters. In another method, we used final resolution correction factors obtained by an independent Monte Carlo method [19]. Time activity curves are then corrected before any fitting of the data to the model.

ASSESSMENT OF MYOCARDIAL PERFUSION RESERVE

Assessment of perfusion at rest and after an hyperemic stimulus such as intravenous dipyridamole or adenosine or after a physiologic stimulus such as exercise has been used to define myocardial perfusion reserve. The basic concept is to quantify the ability of the coronary microvasculature to dilate and the vasodilator reserve is expressed as the ratio of maximal to baseline blood flow [29-32]. This vasodilator reserve is considered to be the best predictor of the functional significance of a coronary lesion. Because of its quantitative capabilities, PET can provide us not only with a ratio of perfusion in the abnormal area over the perfusion in the remote area (similar to the relative ratio obtained with ^{201}Tl imaging), but also a ratio of flow in the abnormal area after vasodilation over the flow in the same area at rest [33]. This latter ratio can be obtained also with the Doppler catheter in the catheterization laboratory but then only velocities and not flow are measured. Furthermore, flow ratios (abnormal area over remote area) as measured by ^{201}Tl or [^{99m}Tc]Methoxy-isobuthyl-isonitrile significantly underestimate the magnitude of the flow disparity between stenotic and normal perfusion beds during vasodilation [34] and, therefore, estimates of absolute perfusion with appropriate tracer kinetics modelling would offer the best approximation of transmural perfusion reserve in patients.

Normal volunteers. Absolute regional myocardial perfusion has been estimated both at rest and during coronary vasodilation in 187 healthy humans in different centres, using PET with both [^{13}N]ammonia [35-39] and [^{15}O]water [11,12,40-43]. The myocardial blood flow values obtained with [^{15}O]water and [^{13}N]ammonia were similar and comparable rates of normal coronary vasodilation reserve were obtained in studies using adenosine or dipyridamole, ranging between 2.9 and 4.4. The variation in vasodilation response to dipyridamole with values of coronary flow reserve ranging from 1.5 to 6.5 is consistent with previous observation using Doppler catheter measurements of coronary flow velocity and also showed that in many cases standard dose dipyridamole may produce submaximal vasodilation. When the abovementioned normal results are compared to the results obtained from patients with cardiovascular disease, it is important to look at the possible confounding effects of two variables influencing myocardial blood flow, i.e. the rate pressure product and the age. It is important to normalize baseline myocardial blood flow for the oxygen demand or for the rate-pressure product. Also, baseline myocardial blood flow tends to increase linearly with age as a consequence of an age related increase in cardiac work [39] and additionally, a reduction in hyperemic flow in subjects older than 60 years has been reported [42,44]. Both mechanisms will contribute to reduce the calculated flow reserve with age.

Coronary artery disease. The relationship between stenosis severity measured by coronary angiography and regional myocardial perfusion was assessed by PET with [^{15}O]water [45], [^{13}N]ammonia [46,47] and ^{82}Rb [48]. In humans, resting myocardial blood flow is preserved even with up to 95% stenosis of a coronary artery [45]. The hyperemic response to dipyridamole and adenosine becomes attenuated at greater than 40% diameter stenosis and is abolished at greater than 80% stenosis [45-47]. Although the inverse relation between stenosis severity and coronary vasodilator reserve was highly significant, a certain degree of variability was observed mainly for stenosis of intermediate severity. However, variability was less when minimal coronary resistance was plotted against stenosis severity indicating the importance of accounting for interindividual differences in perfusion pressure [45]. The relationship between regional perfusion and regional wall motion assessed by echocardiography has been investigated with [^{13}N]ammonia following dipyridamole infusion [49]. Dipyridamole flow in regions subtended by stenotic vessels was lower in the presence of inducible wall motion abnormality (1.1 ± 0.3 ml/min/g) compared to regions without dysfunction (2.0 ± 0.4 ml/min/g, p<0.01).

Table 2. Regional myocardial perfusion reserve in CAD patients assessed with [^{15}O]water and PET

% area stenosis	normal	40-59%	60-79%	≥ 80%
Resting MBF (ml/min/100g)	94±28	127±52	116±43	123±50
Adenosine/dipyridamole MBF	344±147	207±83	151±37	122±36
CFR	3.7±1.2	1.9±1.1	1.6±0.9	1.1±0.3

MBF : myocardial blood flow (mL.min^{-1}.100g^{-1})
CFR : coronary flow reserve (from reference 45)

Table 3. Regional myocardial perfusion reserve in CAD patients assessed with [^{13}N]ammonia and PET

% area stenosis	normal	50-75%	57-95%	95-100%
Resting MBF (ml/min/100g)	71±15	69±1	57±23	58±7
Adenosine MBF	203±62	148±42	115±44	79±18
CFR	2.9±0.7	2.2±0.5	2.1±0.5	1.4±0.3

MBF : myocardial blood flow (mL.min^{-1}.100g^{-1})
CFR : coronary flow reserve (from reference 46)

The effect of PTCA on coronary flow reserve was studied in patients with single vessel CAD and chronic stable angina without a previous myocardial infarction. Coronary flow reserve in the distribution territory of the lesioned artery was shown to recover only gradually in the 3 months after the intervention [50]. The coronary vasodilator response in the region subtended by the previously stenosed coronary artery was impaired for the first 24 hours after angioplasty because of an increase in basal coronary blood flow and a reduction in the maximal vasodilator response. At 7 days, it was still impaired because of an increase in basal coronary blood flow although the maximal blood flow response to dipyridamole has returned to normal. By contrast, Walsh et al. [51] used PET to measure the coronary vasodilator response after angioplasty and reported that it returned to normal in all patients after the procedure but this study was limited because individual patients were studied at different time intervals (range 1 to 18) days after angioplasty with no serial studies. In studies using ^{201}Tl stress imaging, this delay in the recovery of perfusion has also being reported in patients persisting between 4 and 18 days after angioplasty.

Measurements of perfusion in remote normally contracting myocardium supplied by angiographically normal coronary arteries in patients with a significant CAD elsewhere, have shown that the absolute values of flow after vasodilation were significantly lower than those measured in normals [36,52,53]. Although most studies in larger patient populations compared with age-matched controls are needed, it can be speculated that a chronic increase in the loading conditions of remote myocardium may result in structural remodelling of the vascular tree, as seen in arterial hypertension. Alternatively, angiographically undetectable atherosclerosis could result in endothelial dysfunction which could be responsible for a blunted flow reserve. After myocardial infarction, similar to the findings in patients with chronic angina, coronary flow reserve in the remote region was also found to be abnormal initially and to improve at 6 months [54].

Myocardial perfusion has also been measured in patients with chest pain, ischemic-like stress ECG and angiographically normal coronary arteries (syndrome X). When patients with syndrome X are compared with control subjects, no differences are found in myocardial perfusion either at rest or after pharmacological stress, despite syndrome X patients experiencing chest pain after dipyridamole to the same extent as patients with CAD. These findings, together with the absence of any relation among myocardial perfusion, chest pain, and ECG changes under stress, further cast doubts on ischemia as the basis of the reported chest pain, at least in the majority of these patients [55].

Progression and regression of coronary artery disease. Assessment of myocardial perfusion reserve can identify early atherosclerosis in asymptomatic subjects at a high risk for CAD. A study compared age-matched patients with a strong family history of premature CAD with a second group of asymptomatic male subjects without risk factors for CAD [56]. It was shown that coronary flow reserve was significantly lower in the patients with high risk and the degree of impaired flow reserve correlated with the severity of lipid abnormality. These data suggest a potential application of myocardial perfusion measurements in the early detection of CAD in high-risk populations. Moreover, the monitoring of flow reserve could serve as a useful end-point in the assessment of therapy designed to prevent the progression of CAD. The size and severity of myocardial perfusion abnormalities by PET after dipyridamole stress have been shown to decrease or improve in patients undergoing intense dietary changes and treatment with cholesterol-lowering drugs in comparison to a worsening in patients treated with standard antianginal therapy alone [57,58].

Conclusions

Measurements of regional myocardial perfusion at rest and after vasodilation using PET have provided the means to evaluate the functional significance of epicardial coronary stenosis in patients. Improved diagnostic accuracy is obtained with PET as compared to

SPET in evaluating patients with known or suspected CAD. The major advantage of PET is its ability to give attenuation -corrected images which increases the specificity of the diagnostic test. In addition to the diagnostic evaluation of CAD, myocardial perfusion imaging with PET can provide quantitative assessment of myocardial blood flow. This quantitative assessment of myocardial coronary flow reserve allows a physiologic characterization of CAD.

Acknowledgements

This work was supported in part by a Research Concerted Action grant 91/96-146 and from an EEC Concerted Action on PET investigation

References

1. Bonow RO, Berman DS, Gibbons RJ, et al. Cardiac positron emission tomography: a report for health professionals from the committee on advanced cardiac imaging and technology of the council on clinical cardiology, American Heart Association. 1991;84:447-54.
2. Schelbert H, et al. Position statement: clinical use of cardiac positron emission tomography. Position paper of the cardiovascular council of the Society of Nuclear Medicine. J Nucl Med 1993;34:1385-88.
3. Ritchie JL, Bateman TM, Bonow RO, et al. Guidelines for clinical use of cardiac radionuclide imaging: report of the American College of Cardiology/American Heart Association task force on assessment of diagnostic and therapeutic cardiovascular procedures (Committee on Radionuclide Imaging), developed in collaboration with the American Society of Nuclear Cardiology. J Am Coll Cardiol 1995;25:521-47.
4. Schelbert H, Wisenberg G, Phelps ME, et al. Non-invasive assessment of coronary stenoses by myocardial imaging during pharmacologic coronary vasodilation. VI. Detection of coronary artery disease in man with intravenous N-13 ammonia and positron computed tomography. Am J Cardiol 1982;49:1197-207.
5. Demer LL, Gould KL, Goldstein RA, et al. Assessment of coronary artery disease severity by positron emission tomography. Comparison with quantitative arteriography in 193 patients. Circulation 1989;79:825-35.
6. Tamaki N, Yonekura Y, Senda M, et al. Value and limitation of stress thallium-201 single photon emission computed tomography: comparison with nitrogen-13 ammonia positron tomography. J Nucl Med 1988;29:1181-88.
7. Go R, Marwick T, McIntyre W, et al. A prospective comparison of rubidium-82 PET and thallium-201 SPECT myocardial perfusion imaging utilizing a single dipyridamole stress in the diagnosis of coronary artery disease. J Nucl Med 1990;31:1899-905.
8. Stewart R, Schwaiger M, Molina E, et al. Comparison of rubidium-82 positron emission tomography and thallium-201 SPECT imaging for detection of coronary artery disease. Am J Cardiol 1981;48:1077-85.
9. Patterson RE, Eisner RL, Horowitz SF. Comparison of cost-effectiveness and utility of exercise ECG, single photon emission computed tomography, positron emission tomography, and coronary angiography for diagnosis of coronary artery disease. Circulation 1995;91:54-65.
10. Bergmann SR, Fox KAA, Rand AL, et al. Quantification of regional myocardial blood flow in vivo with $H_2{}^{15}O$. Circulation 1984;70:724-33.

11. Bergmann SR, Herrero P, Markham J, Weinheimer CJ, Walsh MN. Non-invasive quantification of myocardial blood flow in human subjects with O-15 labelled water and positron emission tomography. J Am Coll Cardiol 1989;14:639-52.
12. Araujo LI, Lammertsma AA, Rhodes CG, et al. Non-invasive quantification of regional myocardial blood flow in normal volunteers and patients with coronary artery disease using oxygen-15 labeled carbon dioxide inhalation and positron emission tomography. Circulation 1991;83:875-85.
13. Bol A, Melin JA, Vanoverschelde J-L, et al. Direct comparison of [^{13}N]ammonia and [^{15}O] water estimates of perfusion with quantification of regional myocardial blood flow by microspheres. Circulation 1993;87:512-25.
14. Muzik O, Beanlands RSB, Hutchins GD, Mangner TJ, Nguyen N, Schwaiger M. Validation of nitrogen-13 ammonia tracer kinetic model for quantification of myocardial blood flow using PET. J Nucl Med 1993;34:83-91.
15. Kuhle WG, Porenta G, Huang SC, et al. Quantification of regional myocardial blood flow using 13N-ammonia and reoriented dynamic positron emission tomographic imaging. Circulation 1992;86:1004-17.
16. Herrero P, Markham J, Shelton ME, Bergmann SR. Implementation and evaluation of a two-compartment model for quantification of myocardial perfusion with rubidium-82 and positron emission tomography. Circ Res 1992;70:496-507.
17. Henes CG, Bergmann SR, Perez JE, Sobel BE, Geltman EM. The time course of restoration of nutritive perfusion, myocardial oxygen consumption, and regional function after coronary thrombolysis. Cor Art Dis 1990;1:687-96.
18. Czernin J, Porenta G, Brunken R, et al. Regional blood flow, oxidative metabolism, and glucose utilization in patients with recent myocardial infarction. Circulation 1993;88:884-95.
19. Vanoverschelde J-L, Melin JA, Bol A, et al. Regional oxidative metabolism in patients after recovery from reperfused anterior myocardial infarction. Circulation 1992;85:9-21.
20. Gewirtz H, Fischman AJ, Abraham S, Gilson M, Strauss HW, Alpert NM. Positron emission tomographic measurements of absolute regional myocardial blood flow permits identification of non-viable myocardium in patients with chronic myocardial infarction. J Am Coll Cardiol 1994;23:851-59.
21. Piérard LA, DeLandsheere CM, Berthe C, Rigo P, Kulbertus HE. Identification of viable myocardium by echocardiography during dobutamine infusion in patients with myocardial infarction after thrombolytic therapy: comparison with positron emission tomography. J Am Coll Cardiol 1990;15:1021-31.
22. Depré C, Vanoverschelde J-L, Melin JA, et al. Structural and metabolic correlates of the reversibility of chronic left ventricular ischemic dysfunction in humans. Am J Physiol 1995;268:in press.
23. Grandin C, Wijns W, Melin JA, et al. Delineation of myocardial viability with positron emission tomography: incremental value of quantitative flow and metabolic assessment for identification of reversible dysfunction after coronary revascularization. J Nucl Med 1995, in press.
24. Wijns W, Vanoverschelde J-L, Gerber B, et al. Evidence that myocardial stunning occurs in humans following unstable angina. J Am Coll Cardiol 1995:427A.
25. Rahimtoola SH. The hibernating myocardium. Am Heart J 1989;117:211-21.
26. Vanoverschelde J-L, Wijns W, Depré C, et al. Mechanisms of chronic regional postischemic dysfunction in humans: new insights from the study of non-infarcted collateral dependent myocardium. Circulation 1993;87:1513-23.
27. Shen Y-T, Vatner SF. Mechanism of impaired myocardial function during progressive coronary stenosis in conscious pigs: hibernation versus stunning. Circ Res 1995;76:479-88.
28. Parodi O, Schelbert HR, Schwaiger M, Hansen H, Selin C, Hoffman EJ. Cardiac emission computed tomography: underestimation of regional tracer concentrations due to wall motion abnormalities. J Comput Assist Tomography 1984;8:1083-92.

29. Gould KL, Lipscomb K, Hamilton GW. A physiologic basis for assessing critical coronary stenosis: instantaneaous flow response and regional distribution during coronary hyperemia as measures of coronary flow reserve. Am J Cardiol 1974;33:87-94.
30. Gould KL. Non-invasive assessment of coronary stenoses by myocardial imaging during coronary vasodilation, I: physiologic principles and experimental validation. Am J Cardiol 1978;41:267-78.
31. Hoffman JIE. Maximal coronary flow and the concept of coronary vascular reserve. Circulation 1984;70:153-59.
32. Klocke FJ. Measurements of coronary flow reserve: defining pathophysiology versus making decisions about patient care. Circulation 1987;76:1183-89.
33. De Silva R, Camici PG. Role of positron emission tomography in the investigation of human coronary circulatory function. Cardiovasc Res 1994;28:1595-1612.
34. Glover DK, Ruiz M, Edwards NC, et al. Comparison between 201TI and 99mTc sestamibi uptake during adenosine-induced vasodilation as a function of coronary stenosis severity. Circulation 1995;91:813-20.
35. Camici P, Chiriatti G, Lorenzoni R, et al. Coronary vasodilation is impaired in both hypertrophied and non-hypertrophied myocardium of patients with hypertrophic cardiomyopathy: a study with nitrogen-13 ammonia and positron emission tomography. J Am Coll Cardiol 1991;17:879-86.
36. Sambuceti G, Parodi O, Marcassa C, et al. Alteration in regulation of myocardial blood flow in one vessel coronary artery disease determined by positron emission tomography. Am J Cardiol 1993;72:538-43.
37. Chan SY, Brunken RC, Czernin J, et al. Comparison of maximal myocardial blood flow during adenosine infusion with that of intravenous dipyridamole in normal men. J Am Coll Cardiol 1992;20:979-85.
38. Muzik O, Beanlands R, Wolfe E, Hutchins GD, Schwaiger M. Automated region definition for cardiac Nitrogen-13-ammonia PET imaging. J Nucl Med 1993;34:336-44.
39. Czernin J, Muller P, Chan S, et al. Influence of age and haemodynamics on myocardial blood flow and flow reserve. Circulation 1993;88:62-9.
40. Geltman EM, Henes CG, Senneff MJ, Sobel BE, Bergmann SR. Increased myocardial perfusion at rest and diminished perfusion reserve in patients with angina and angiographically normal coronary arteries. J Am Coll Cardiol 1990;16:586-95.
41. Merlet P, Mazoyer B, Hittinger L, et al. Assessment of coronary reserve in man: comparison between positron emission tomography with oxygen-15 labelled water and intracoronary Doppler technique. J Nucl Med 1993;34:1899-1904.
42. Uren NG, Camici PG, Wijns W, et al. The effect of ageing on coronary flow reserve in man. Circulation 1993;88:I-171.
43. Radvan J, Camici PG, Marwick T, Boyd H, Sheridan DJ. Physiological hypertrophy does not affect coronary flow reserve in man. Circulation 1993;88:I-214.
44. Senneff MJ, Geltman EM, Bergmann SR, Hartmann J. Non-invasive delineation of the effects of moderate ageing on myocardial perfusion. J Nucl Med 1991;32:2037-42.
45. Uren NG, Melin JA, De Bruyne B, Wijns W, Baudhuin T, Camici PG. Myocardial blood flow as a function of coronary stenosis severity in man. N Engl J Med 1994;330:1782-88.
46. Beanlands RSB, Muzik O, Sutor R, et al. Noninvasive determination of regioal perfusion reserve in coronary artery disease using N-13 ammonia PET. J Nuc Med 1992;33:826.
47. Di Carli M, Czernin J, Sherman T, et al. Relationship between stenosis severity, hyperemic blood flow, flow reserve, and coronary resistance in CAD patients. Circulation 1993;88:I-647.

48. Goldstein RA, Kirkeeide RL, Demer LL, et al. Relation between geometric dimensions of coronary artery stenoses and myocardial perfusion reserve in man. J Clin Invest 1987;79:1473-78.
49. Picano E, Parodi E, Lattanzi F, et al. Assessment of anatomic and physiologic severity of single vessel coronary artery lesions by dipyridamole echocardiography: comparison with positron emission tomography and quantitative arteriography. Circulation 1994;89:753-61.
50. Uren NG, Crake T, Lefroy DC, De Silva R, Davies GJ, Maseri A. Delayed recovery of coronary resistive vessel function after coronary angioplasty. J Am Coll Cardiol 1993;21:612-21.
51. Walsh MN, Geltman EM, Steele RL, et al. Augmented myocardial perfusion reserve after coronary angioplasty quantified by positron emission tomography with $H_2{}^{15}O$. J Am Coll Cardiol 1990;15:119-127.
52. Uren NG, Marraccini P, Gistri R, De Silva R, Camici PG. Altered coronary vasodilator reserve and metabolism in myocardium subtended by normal arteries in patients with coronary artery disease. J Am Coll Cardiol 1993;22:650-58.
53. Sambuceti G, Marzullo P, Giorgetti A, et al. Global alteration in perfusion response to increasing oxygen consumption in patients with single-vessel coronary artery disease. Circulation 1994;90:1696-1705.
54. Uren NG, Crake T, Lefroy DC, De Silva R, Davies GJ, Maseri A. Reduced coronary vasodilator function in infarcted and normal myocardium after myocardial infarction. N Engl J Med 1994;331:222-27.
55. Rosen SD, Uren NG, Kaski JC, Tousoulis D, Davies GJ, Camici PG. Coronary vasodilator reserve, pain perception, and sex in patients with syndrome X. Circulation 1994;90:50-60.
56. Dayanikli F, Grambow D, Muzik O, Mosca L, Rubenfire M, Schwaiger M. Early detection of abnormal coronary flow reserve in asymptomatic men at high risk for coronary artery disease using positron emission tomography. Circulation 1994;90:808-17.
57. Gould KL, Martucci JP, Goldberg DI, et al. Short-term cholesterol lowering decreases size and severity of perfusion abnormalities by positron emission tomography after dipyridamole in patients with coronary artery disease : a potential noninvasive marker of healing coronary endothelium. Circulation 1994;89:1530-38.
58. Gould KL. Reversal of coronary atherosclerosis. Clinical promise as the basis for noninvasive management of coronary artery disease. Circulation 1994;90:1558-71.

ASSESSMENT OF MYOCARDIAL VIABILITY WITH PET

3

Juergen vom Dahl

Less than 20 years ago, contractile dysfunction of the myocardium in the distribution territory of a stenosed coronary artery was thought to represent either irreversible damage of myocytes due to myocardial infarction and necrosis, or the effects of transient ischemia. However, during the last decade, experimental and clinical studies demonstrated that regional contractile dysfunction may also occur in the absence of myocardial infarction and may persist for a long time after cessation of ischemia with spontaneous normalization of function. Regional dysfunction in viable myocardium may be either temporary and spontaneously reversible following early reperfusion of a previously occluded vessel (myocardial "stunning" [1]) or sustained in the presence of chronic resting hypoperfusion and potentially reversible following restoration of blood flow by coronary revascularization (myocardial "hibernation" [2]).

The need for non-invasive techniques to specifically identify dysfunctioning but viable and, thus, potentially salvageable myocardium is well appreciated, since angiographic evaluation of regional contractility and epicardial coronary perfusion does not distinguish between viable myocardium and irreversibly damaged tissue. Positron emission tomography (PET) imaging in combination with various tracers allows to detect changes that occur at the cellular level and, thus, permits evaluation of tissue viability on the basis of myocardial perfusion, cell membrane integrity, and metabolic activity. Worldwide, approximately 200 PET facilities [3], most of them located in the United States, Japan, and Germany, perform cardiac studies with the main indication being assessment of myocardial viability in patients with coronary artery disease and left ventricular dysfunction.

This review focuses on the clinical application of different PET imaging approaches for the assessment of myocardial viability.

PET Imaging Of Mycardial Perfusion And Metabolism

Because impairment of mechanical function reflects abnormalities in myocardial metabolism, PET has been used to identify metabolic processes that may differentiate viable from nonviable myocardium. The currently most widespread used PET approach in clinical practice is the combined evaluation of myocardial perfusion using N-13 labeled ammonia, O-15 labeled water, or rubidium-82, and myocardial metabolism. Particularly, 2-[^{18}F]fluoro-2-deoxy-D-glucose ([^{18}F]FDG) is widely used for the non-invasive assessment of exogeneous glucose utilization, since metabolic changes

R. Bares and G. Lucignani (eds.) Clinical PET, 25–34.

associated with myocardial ischemia have been well-defined and the favourable physical characteristics of [^{18}F]FDG with a half-life of 110 minutes provide good image quality using static imaging without the absolute need for quantification and dynamic imaging. [^{18}F]FDG is a glucose analogue that reflects transmembraneous transport and hexokinase-mediated phosphorylation of glucose by the myocyte. Myocardial metabolism in ischemic myocardium is characterized by impaired oxidation of fatty acids, accelerated glycogen breakdown, and increased glycolytic flux [4]. Based on experimental data in animals, markedly decreased [^{18}F]FDG uptake has been proven as a marker of irreversible myocardial damage, whereas maintained or elevated [^{18}F]FDG uptake has been proposed as a marker of preserved tissue viability in segments with chronic hypoperfusion. This concept of perfusion metabolism mismatch, introduced by Marshall et al. [5], has been employed to evaluate the predictive value of [^{18}F]FDG uptake for functional tissue recovery after revascularization. Tillisch et al. [6] demonstrated for the first time, that asynergic areas of preserved [^{18}F]FDG uptake are most likely to improve functionally, whereas those with absent or low [^{18}F]FDG uptake are unlikely to recover following coronary revascularization. This landmark study has been followed by several subsequent reports confirming the high predictive accuracy of PET imaging for postrevascularization outcome in regional and global left ventricular function using this match / mismatch concept (Table 1) [7-12]. Interestingly, and of significant clinical impact, studies focusing on patients with markedly reduced ejection fraction demonstrated not only significant improvement of regional but, more important perhaps, of global left ventricular function, indicating that this patient population may be the one benefitting most from PET viability imaging [6, 10, 12, 13]. These findings are not only of clinical but also of economic importance, since treatment planning in ischemic heart failure (coronary revascularization vs heart transplantation or medical treatment) can be optimized and unnecessary costly procedures probably avoided.

However, as can been appreciated from Table 1, the number of subjects preoperatively evaluated by PET imaging is still relatively small, even after addition of those studies with single photon emission tomography (SPET) perfusion imaging and PET metabolic imaging as presented in Table 2.

Furthermore, these studies have been performed using different patient subgroups (e.g. mild or severe left ventricular function), different metabolic conditions during [^{18}F]FDG imaging (oral glucose loading or fasting), and various diagnostic modalities to evaluate functional outcome (echocardiography, radionuclide ventriculography, left ventricular angiography) with mostly qualitative assessment of regional contractility (visual scoring). A large prospective study with treatment blinded to preoperative nuclear imaging results and well defined viability by quantitative thresholds of functional improvement has not been carried out yet (but may be ethically difficult to justify).

PET imaging of myocardial perfusion and metabolism also enables identification of patients at high risk for future cardiac events such as myocardial infarction, emergency revascularization, cardiac arrest, or cardiac death. Studies from the Universities at Michigan, Los Angeles, and Kyoto demonstrated that patients with evidence for ischemically compromized myocardium are at high risk for future cardiac events if not revascularized [14-16]. On the other hand, revascularization of myocardium identified as mostly irreversibly damaged by PET, did not result in significant prognostic benefits as compared to medical treatment.

There are several limitations associated with [^{18}F]FDG imaging. Patients with acute or early after acute myocardial infarction are often under heparin treatment following thrombolytic therapy or present with high levels of plasma catecholamines, both factors that suppress cardiac glucose utilization and [^{18}F]FDG uptake [17,18]. However, despite these potential limitations, [^{18}F]FDG imaging in patients with acute or recent myocardial infarction has been shown to provide similar prognostic information regarding myocardial viability and the potential of functional improvement during follow-up [19, 20].

Table 1. Studies with preoperative evaluation of myocardial viability by PET perfusion/metabolism imaging and with functional evaluation following coronary revascularization.

Author	Pts	Segm	+ PV %	- PV %	Comments
Tillisch [6]	17	67	88	92	
Tamaki [7]	22	46	78	78	fasting protocol
Marwick [9]	16	85	68	79	post exercise
Carrel [10]	23	68	84	75	angiographic follow-up
Gropler [11]	34	116	52	81	all regions
		57	72	82	regions with severe dysfunction
Tamaki [47]	31	76	79	91	fasting, quantitative analysis
vom Dahl [12]	37	191	48	85	all regions
		35	88	86	regions with severe dysfunction
Total	180	649	71 (79)	83 (85)	

Pts: number of patients studied.
Segm: number of revascularized segments.
+ PV: positive predictive value (%).
- PV: negative predictive value (%).

The hormonal and metabolic milieu influences myocardial glucose and, thus, [^{18}F]FDG uptake as well as [^{18}F]FDG clearance from the blood by other glucose utilizing tissue [21]. Particularly, patients with abnormal glucose tolerance or diabetes mellitus are at higher risk of [^{18}F]FDG studies of limited quality due to suppressed [^{18}F]FDG uptake of the myocardium. Whereas recent studies demonstrated significant improvement of image quality by adequate supplementation of insulin prior to [^{18}F]FDG injection and during imaging, even by use of an euglycemic-hyperinsulinemic clamping technique [22, 23], there is ongoing controversy concerning the most suitable and clinically useful imaging protocol (glucose loading, fasting, clamping) [24, 25]. Furthermore, regional heterogeneity of myocardial substrate utilization, especially under fasting conditions, with overestimation of ischemic myocardium and low [^{18}F]FDG uptake in normally perfused regions influences the visual interpretation of cardiac PET studies [26, 27]. If quantitative measurements of myocardial glucose utilization or normalization of individual [^{18}F]FDG uptake to the region with normal or best perfusion, as suggested by several groups [28, 29] will resolve these problems remains open and has to be clarified in future studies. These briefly outlined factors are ongoing challenges for the optimization of [^{18}F]FDG imaging procedures.

Despite these limitations, PET imaging of myocardial perfusion and metabolism using [^{18}F]FDG today represents the most sensitive method to characterize myocardial viability and has been accepted as the non-invasive "gold-standard". Other techniques such as stress echocardiography or myocardial scintigraphy using Tl-201 chloride with reinjction protocols or the newer Tc-99m based tracers (probably in the near future with tissue attenuation correction) have to be compared with this PET approach for their clinical value.
Emerging approaches for the assessment of myocardial viability using PET technology include the water-perfusable tissue index, the rubidium uptake and retention approach, quantitative measurements of myocardial blood flow, and the assessment of oxidative metabolism with C-11 acetate.

The Water-Perfusable Tissue Index (PTI)

The PTI is defined as the proportion of the total anatomical tissue within a given region of interest that is capable of rapidly exchanging water and has units g (perfusable tissue/g (total anatomic tissue). The fraction of extravascular tissue density that can be perfused with O-15 labeled water represents myocardium capable of maintaining transmembraneous ion concentration gradients, which is presumed to indicate preserved tissue viability. In contrast, scar tissue does not exchange water rapidly. After measurements of overall tissue densities by obtaining a transmission scan, calculation of PTI employs PET with O-15 labeled water to measure the exchangeable intracellular water space, and O-15 labeled carbon monoxide to correct for blood pool activity [30]. This approach has been validated in normal volunteers and recently been proposed in patients with coronary artery disease [31, 32]. In 11 patients studied early after a successfully thrombolysed myocardial infarction, dysfunctional segments demonstrating functional improvement displayed a PTI of 0.9±0.1 which was not different from normal tissue. Conversely, despite similar myocardial blood flow at baseline, nonrecovery regions had a PTI of 0.5±0.1. By direct comparison to conventional flow-metabolism PET imaging in 15 patients with old myocardial infarction, regions with a metabolism-flow ratio 1.2 (indicating reversible damage) displayed a PTI of 0.7±0.1 as compared to 0.5±0.1 in regions with a metabolism-flow ratio <1.2 [31]. Similarly, in 12 patients with chronic coronary artery disease and old myocardial infarction who underwent coronary revascularization, PTI was significantly higher (1.0±0.1) in regions with functional recovery at follow-up and was 0.7 in all cases, whereas in nonrecovery regions PTI was always <0.7 (0.6±0.1) [32].
Thus PTI appears to discriminate reliably between reversible and irreversible contractile dysfunction and the authors propose a value of 0.7 (indicating 70% perfused and viable or 30% nonperfused and necrotic tissue) as the critical threshold. However, these promising data have been obtained in a small number of patients only and have to be confirmed in larger patient populations with advanced coronary artery disease and severely depressed left ventricular function. Furthermore, since PTI measures a fraction within a given region, this index does not distinguish between normal and ischemically compromised tissue (which can coexist within a myocardial region) , which is critical for the potential functional recovery. Thus, the clinical impact of this elegant approach has to be awaited.

Quantitative Measurements Of Myocardial Blood Flow

Very recently, PET measurements of absolute regional myocardial blood flow using PET in conjunction with a mathematical model of N-13 labeled ammonia tracer kinetics in 26 patients with chronic myocardial infarction were compared with regional [^{18}F]FDG uptake and correlated to regional wall motion and coronary anatomy [33]. A basal regional blood flow of <0.25 ml/g/min indicated the absence of viable tissue (as demonstrated from dyskinetic wall motion and concordant [^{18}F]FDG uptake reduction) whereas in regions with only mild hypokinesia or normal wall motion (indicating preserved viability) flow was 0.8±0.3 ml/min/g and was 0.39 ml/g/min in 96% of regions. However, since the issue of viability is not critical in normal or only mild hypokinetic contracting myocardium, the question of a lower threshold of perfusion to maintain cell membrane integrity and the potential of functional recovery has still to be answered.

The Rubidium Uptake And Retention Approach

Experimental and preliminary clinical data indicate the usefulness of ^{82}Rb in combination with PET imaging techniques to assess myocardial viability. Like the cationic thallium ions, Rb^+ can substitute for potassium at the sodium pump. Viable myocytes actively transport rubidium cations into the cell, where they are retained. Thus, ^{82}Rb uptake and retention indicates maintained cell membrane integrity. Animal models with coronary occlusion and reperfusion demonstrated rapid ^{82}Rb leakage from irreversibly injured tissue, while the tracer was retained in reversibly damaged and viable tissue [34, 35]. Based on these experimental data, Gould subsequently proposed ^{82}Rb imaging early and late after tracer injection as a new clinical PET approach for definition of tissue viability in patients with previous myocardial infarction [36]. The results were in good correlation to [^{18}F]FDG uptake data obtained in these patients. Recently, the clinical long-term follow-up of 35 patients studied by this approach has been reported and demonstrated its diagnostic value in identifying patients with poor prognosis and those who might benefit from coronary revascularization [37]. Similar preliminary results have been reported using dynamic PET imaging and ^{82}Rb in 27 patients with coronary artery disease [38]. The ^{82}Rb tissue half-time of ischemically compromized tissue with maintained [^{18}F]FDG uptake was significantly higher (75±9 seconds) as compared to regions with markedly reduced [^{18}F]FDG uptake indicating necrosis (57±12 seconds). The main advantage of these interesting approaches is the possibility to perform perfusion and viability studies with one single tracer injection without the need for an on-site cyclotron. However, although comparisons to the [^{18}F]FDG approach have been encouraging, the validation of the rudidium uptake and retention approach by postrevascularization functional assessment has not been reported yet.

C-11 Labeled Acetate

C-11 labeled acetate traces the tricarboxylic acid cycle and has been shown to be closely correlated to oxidative metabolism and, thus, to be a marker of myocardial oxygen consumption. From dynamic PET sequences, oxygen consumption is calculated from myocardial tissue clearance rates of C-11 acetate [39-41]. PET viability imaging using C-11 acetate is based on the assumption that sustained oxygen metabolism is mandatory for cellular survival. In patients studied early after successful thrombolytic therapy for myocardial infarction, functional recovery was associated with improvement of oxidative metabolism as demonstrated by sequential PET studies [42]. In patients with chronic stable coronary artery disease undergoing coronary revascularization, functional recovery was dependent of the preoperative maintenance of oxidative metabolism [43, 44]. A study comparing estimates of myocardial oxidative metabolism by PET and C-11 acetate with glucose metabolism assessed by [^{18}F]FDG uptake in 34 patients demonstrated slightly higher predictive values for the C-11 acetate approach (positive 67%, negative 89%) as compared to [^{18}F]FDG (52% and 81% resp.), with diagnostic accuracy more pronounced in severely dysfunctioning regions (positive: C-11 acetate 85%, [^{18}F]FDG 72%; negative: C-11 acetate 87%, [^{18}F]FDG 82%) [11]. Although this approach is very promising, additional investigations have to be performed in patients with markedly depressed left ventricular function, since they will be the patient population in the future that could benefit most from PET imaging.

Perfusion Imaging Using SPET: The "Hybrid Approach"

Several groups have now performed studies using SPET with Tc-99m isonitriles or Tl-201 chloride as perfusion tracers in combination with PET imaging of [^{18}F]FDG-uptake.

Table 2. Studies with preoperative evaluation of myocardial viability by SPET perfusion and PET metabolism.

Author	Pts	Segm	+ PV %	- PV %	Comments
Lucignani [45]	14	70	79-96	87	[^{99m}Tc]MIBI/[^{18}F]FDG wall motion by RNV
Knuuti [28]	48	90	54	100	[^{99m}TC]MIBI or ^{201}Tl and [^{18}F]FDG wall motion by RNV
			100	100	regions with reduced perfusion
vom Dahl [46]	52	95	52	93	[^{99m}TC]MIBI/[^{18}F]FDG wall motion by quantitative angiographic follow-up
			68	93	successfully revascularized
Total	114	255	65 (87)	94 (94)	

Pts: number of patients studied.
Segm: number of revascularized segments.
+ PV: positive predictive value (%).
- PV: negative predictive value (%).

One rationale for this approach is the lack of availability of an on-site cyclotron for production of positron emitting isotopes. The long physical half-life of [^{18}F]FDG allows transport of the tracer from a central cyclotron to several distant PET scanners, as proposed by the "Satellite concept" in Germany. Sophisticated software allows semiquantitative analysis of tracer uptake from both data sets using SPET and PET. Despite the theoretical disadvantage of missing tissue attenuation correction with SPET, the predictive accuracy of this approach is similar to that of PET imaging of both perfusion and metabolism (Table 2) [28, 45, 46].

Conclusions And Clinical Implications

PET imaging techniques provide several approaches to the noninvasive assessment of myocardial viability in patients with depressed regional or global left ventricular function. The differentiation between irreversibly damaged myocardium and ischemically jeopardized and potentially salvageable tissue with its high diagnostic accuracy influences more and more therapeutic strategies in patients with advanced coronary artery disease. Furthermore, PET viability imaging has proved useful for identification of high-risk patients as well as of those patients who will benefit most from revascularization in terms of improving left ventricular function, reducing symptoms of heart failure, and improving prognosis. However, due to financial considerations, PET viability imaging should be reserved for the patient with severe coronary artery disease and depressed function, in whom the PET results might *change* therapy. It is not necessary in patients with only mild contractile dysfunction or evidence for stress induced ischemia in regions with impaired regional wall motion, since these will be mostly viable and amenable to revascularization.

Since PET technology is expensive and not widely available, PET has challenged and challenges other techniques to improve their diagnostic accuracy. The Tl-201 chloride redistribution-reinjection technique in combination with SPET imaging has been proposed as an alternative approach, as this is more widely available. Stress echocardiography and Doppler tissue imaging by ultrasound are other emerging bed-side techniques that might reduce the need for PET. However, prospective studies comparing these techniques with PET in large patient populations have not been performed yet but are neccessary to futher elucidate their individual indications and limitations.

References

1. Bolli R. Myocardial 'stunning' in man. Circulation 1992;86:1671-91.
2. Rahimtoola SH. The hibernating myocardium. Am Heart J 1989;117:211-21.
3. Schelbert HR. Merits and limitations of raduinuclide approaches to viability and future developments. J Nucl Cardiol 1994;1(2/2):86-96.
4. Liedtke AJ. Alterations of carbohydrate and lipid metabolism in the acutely ischemic heart. Prog Cardiovasc Dis 1981;23:321-36.
5. Marshall RC, Tillisch JH, Phelps ME, et al. Identification and differentiation of resting myocardial ischemia in man with positron computed tomography,18F-labeled fluorodeoxyglucose and N-13 ammonia. Circulation 1983;67:766-78.
6. Tillisch J, Brunken R, Marshall R, et al. Reversibility of cardiac wall-motion abnormalities predicted by positron tomography. N Engl J Med 1986;314:884-8.

7. Tamaki N, Yonekura Y, Yamashita K, et al. Positron emission tomography using fluorine-18 deoxyglucose in evaluation of coronary artery bypass grafting. Am J Cardiol 1989;64(14):860-5.
8. Marwick TH, MacIntyre WJ, Nemec JJ, Go RT, Saha GB. Post-Exercise F-18 Deoxyglucose PET predicts functional recovery of hibernating myocardium after revascularization (abstr). Europ Heart J 1991;12(Abstr Suppl):17.
9. Marwick TH, MacIntyre WJ, Lafont A, Nemec JJ, Salcedo EE. Metabolic responses of hibernating and infarcted myocardium to revascularization. Circulation 1992;85:1347-53.
10. Carrel T, Jenni R, Haubold-Reuter S, von Schulthess G, Pasic M, Turina M. Improvement of severely reduced left ventricular function after surgical revascularization in patients with preoperative myocardial infarction. Eur J Cardiothorac Surg 1992;6:479-84.
11. Gropler RJ, Geltman EM, Sampathkumaran K, et al. Comparison of carbon-11-acetate with fluorine-18-fluorodeoxyglucose for delineating viable myocardium by positron emission tomography. J Am Coll Cardiol 1993;22:1587-97.
12. vom Dahl J, Eitzman DT, Al-Aouar ZR, Kanter HL, Hicks RJ, Schwaiger M. Relationship between regional function, perfusion, and metabolism in patients with advanced coronary artery disease undergoing surgical revascularization. Circulation 1994;90:2355-66.
13. Besozzi MC, Brown MD, Hubner KF, et al. Retrospective post therapy evaluation of cardiac function in 208 coronary artery disease patients evaluated by positron emission tomography. J Nucl Med 1992;33:885.
14. Eitzman D, Al-Aouar Z, Kanter HL, et al. Clinical outcome of patients with advanced coronary artery disease after viability studies with positron emission tomography. J Am Coll Cardiol 1992;20:559-65.
15. Tamaki N, Kawamoto M, Takahashi N, et al. Prognostic value of an increase in fluorine-18 deoxyglucose uptake in patients with myocardial infarction: comparison with stress thallium imaging. J Am Coll Cardiol 1993;22:1621-7.
16. DiCarli MF, Davidson M, Little R, et al. Value of metabolic imaging with positron emission tomography for evaluating prognosis in patients with coronary artery disease and left ventricular dysfunction. Am J Cardiol 1994;73:527-33.
17. Wisneski JA, Gertz EW, Neese RA, Gruenke LD, Morris L, Craig JC. Metabolic fate of extracted glucose in normal human myocardium. J Clin Invest 1985;76:1819-27.
18. Merhige ME, Ekas R, Mossberg K, Taegtmeyer H, Gould KL. Catecholamine stimulation, substrate competition, and myocardial glucose uptake in conscious dogs assessed with positron emission tomography. Circ Res 1987;61(suppl II):II 124-9.
19. Schwaiger M, Brunken R, Grover-McKay M, et al. Regional myocardial metabolism in patients with acute myocardial infarction assessed by positron emission tomography. J Am Coll Cardiol 1986;8(800-8).
20. Pierard LA, De Landsheere CM, Berthe C, Rigo P, Kulbertus HE. Identification of viable myocardium by echocardiography during dobutamine infusion in patients with myocardial infarction after thrombolytic therapy: comparison with positron emission tomography. J Am Coll Cardiol 1990;15:1021-31.
21. Berry JJ, Baker JA, Pieper KS, Hanson MW, Hoffman JM, Coleman RE. The effect of metabolic milieu on cardiac PET imaging using fluorine-18-deoxyglucose and nitrogen-13-ammonia in normal volunteers. J Nucl Med 1991;32:1518-25.
22. Knuuti MJ, Nuutila P, U. R, et al. Euglycemic hyperinsulinemic clamp and oral glucose load in stimulating myocardial glucose utilization during positron emission tomography. J Nucl Med 1992;33:1255-62.
23. vom Dahl J, Herman WH, Hicks RJ, et al. Myocardial glucose uptake in patients with insulin-dependent diabetes mellitus assessed quantitatively by dynamic positron emission tomography. Circulation 1993;88:395-404.

24. Schelbert HR. Euglycemic hyperinsulinemic clamp and oral glucose load in stimulating myocardial glucose utilization during positron emission tomography. J Nucl Med 1992;33:1263-66.
25. Tamaki N. Myocardial FDG PET studies with the fasting, oral glucose-loading or insulin clamp methods. J Nucl Med 1992;33:1263-1268.
26. Hicks RJ, Herman WH, Kalff V, et al. Quantitative evaluation of regional substrate metabolism in the human heart by positron emission tomography. J Am Coll Cardiol 1991;18:101-11.
27. Gropler RJ, SiegEl BA, Lee KJ, et al. Nonuniformity in myocardial accumulation of F-18 fluorodeoxyglucose in normal fasted humans. J Nucl Med 1990;31(11):1749-56.
28. Knuuti MJ, Saraste M, Nuutila P, et al. Myocardial viability: fluorine-18-deoxyglucose positron emission tomography in prediction of wall motion recovery after revascularization. Am Heart J 1994;127:785-96.
29. Altehoefer C, vom Dahl J, Biedermann M, et al. Significance of defect severity in Technetium-99m-MIBI SPECT at rest to assess myocardial viability: comparison with Fluorine-18-FDG PET. J Nucl Med 1994;35:569-74.
30. Iida H, Rhodes CG, de Silva R, et al. Myocardial tissue fraction: correction for partial volume effects and measure of tissue viability. J Nucl Med 1991;32:2169-75.
31. Yamamoto Y, de Silva R, Rhodes CG, et al. A new strategy for the assessment of viable myocardium and regional blood flow using O-15 water and dynamic positron emission tomography. Circulation 1992;86:167-78.
32. de Silva R, Yamamoto Y, Rhodes C, et al. Preoperative prediction of the outcome of coronary revascularization using positron emission tomography. Circulation 1992;86:1738-42.
33. Gewirtz H, Fischman AJ, Abraham S, Gilson M, Strauss HW, Alpert NM. Positron emission tomographic measurements of absolute regional myocardial blood flow permits identification of nonviable myocardium in patients with chronic myocardial infarction. J Am Coll Cardiol 1994;23:851-9.
34. Goldstein R. Kinetics of Rubidium-82 after coronary occlusion and reperfusion. Assessment of patency and viability in open-chested dogs. J Clin Invest 1985;75:1131-7.
35. Goldstein RA. Rubidium-82 kinetics after coronary occlusion: Temporal relation of net myocardial accumulation and viability in open-chested dogs. J Nucl Med 1986;27:1456-1461.
36. Gould KL, Yoshida K, Hess MJ, Haynie M, Mullani N, Smalling RW. Myocardial metabolism of fluorodeoxyglucose compared to cell membrane integrity for the potassium analogue rubidium-82 for assessing infarct size in man by PET. J Nucl Med 1991;32:1-9.
37. Yoshida K, Gould KL. Quantitative relation of myocardial infarct size and myocardial viability by positron emission tomography to left ventricular ejection fraction and 3-year mortality with and without revascularization. J Am Coll Cardiol 1993;22:984-97.
38. vom Dahl J, Muzik O, Wolfe ER, Schwaiger M. Rubidium 82 kinetics assessed by positron emission tomography for characterization of myocardial viability (abstr). J Am Coll Cardiol 1992;19:142A.
39. Brown MA, Myears DW, Bergmann SR. Noninvasive assessment of canine myocardial oxidative metabolism with carbon-11 acetate and positron emission tomography. J Am Coll Cardiol 1988;12:1054-1063.
40. Armbrecht JJ, Buxton DB, Schelbert HR. Validation of (1-11C] acetate as a tracer for noninvasive assessment of oxidative metabolism with positron emission tomography in normal, ischemic, postischemic, and hyperemic canine myocardium. Circulation 1990;81:1594-1605.

41. Henes CG, Bergmann SR, Walsh MN, Sobel BE, Geltman EM. Assessment of myocardial oxidative metabolic reserve with positron emission tomography and carbon-11 acetate. J Nucl Med 1989;30:1489-99.
42. Henes CG, Bergmann SR, Perez JE, Sobel BE, Geltman EM. The time course of restoration of nutritive perfusion, myocardial oxygen consumption, and regional function after coronary thrombolysis. Coronary Artery Dis 1990;1:687-96.
43. Gropler RJ, Geltman EM, Sampathkumaran K, et al. Functional recovery after coronary revascularization for chronic coronary artery disease is dependent on maintenance of oxidative metabolism. J Am Coll Cardiol 1992;20:569-77.
44. Gropler RJ, Siegel BA, Sampathkumaran K, et al. Dependence of recovery of contractile function on maintenance of oxidative metabolism after myocardial infarction. J Am Coll Cardiol 1992;19:989-97.
45. Lucignani G, Paolini G, Landoni C, et al. Presurgical identification of hibernating myocardium by combined use of technetium-99m hexakis 2-methoxyisobutylisonitrile single photon emission tomography and fluorine-18 fluoro-2-deoxy-D-glucose positron emission tomography in patients with coronary artery disease. Eur J Nucl Med 1992;19:874-81.
46. vom Dahl J, Altehoefer C, Sheehan FH, et al. Myocardial viability assessed by combined imaging using myocardial scintigraphy and positron emission tomography: impact on treatment and functional outcome following revascularization (abstr). J Am Coll Cardiol 1994;23(Suppl):117A.
47. Tamaki N. Current status of viability assessment with positron emission tomography. J Nucl Cardiol 1994;1:40-7.

Part Two:
PET in Oncology

PET IN ONCOLOGY - CLINICAL DEMANDS

4

Maike de Wit

In industrialized countries the incidence of cancer is steadily increasing and ranks now second as a cause of death. New techniques are therefore needed to optimize diagnosis of malignant disorders. While high resolution computed tomography (CT) and magnetic resonance imaging (MRI) have improved the ability to detect changes in size or shape of physiological structures, it has become even more difficult to judge the significance of such findings.

Main Diagnostic Problems In Clinical Oncology

1. In spite of advanced techniques in CT or MRI, even today the "simple question" whether a lesion is benign or malignant is hard to answer. The different programs currently used for tumor screening produce a growing number of findings of uncertain clinical relevance. Screening for cancer, however, is only useful if definite diagnoses can be established. Examples of such uncertain findings are palpable breast nodules, ambiguous mammographies, or solitary pulmonary nodules detected in the course of preoperative examinations. In case of early stages of malignant disease immediate surgery should be performed using a minimum of diagnostic tests. On the other hand, patients with benign lesions should be spared from the risk and expenses of surgery and invasive diagnostic techniques.
2. Besides detection knowledge about the exact tumor extension, it is essential to select adequate therapeutic strategies. Staging should be as simple as possible, but at the same time as accurate as possible, too. Patients with unresectable or metastatic tumors should not undergo explorative surgery whenever possible. A typical example for this type of disease is prostate cancer with pelvic lymph node metastases.
3. Discrimination between benign and malignant lesions is also a common problem after chemo- or radiotherapy. Residual masses are frequently found and need to be further classified as viable tumor or fibrotic scar. This is especially true for germ cell tumors or lymphomas. In the latter, early discrimation between treatment failure or success is important in order to change the therapeutic strategy if necessary.
4. During follow-up after surgery or radiotherapy (e.g. because of colorectal cancer) it is often uncertain whether local masses are due to fibrotic scars or tumor recurrence.

In oncology new diagnostic methods are only relevant if they contribute to therapeutic decisions. In the following chapters a number of clinical settings, which might benefit from the use of PET, will be discussed in detail.

R. Bares and G. Lucignani (eds.) Clinical PET, 37–44.

Malignant Lymphoma

The incidence of malignant lymphoma seems to be slowly increasing and has now reached approximately 15/100,000/year [1]. Treatment is adjusted to stage and type of disease using radiotherapy or chemotherapy either alone or in combination [2,3]. To keep the rate of relapses and complications low, reliable staging is essential. After a basic program including clinical, in-vitro, radiological, scintigraphic, and histopathological methods more sophisticated additional tests will be performed, if an advanced stage has to be excluded (Table 1). Scintigraphy with ^{67}Gallium-citrate is known to have a high sensitivity and specificity in early stages of disease. However, its predictive value is rather low when evaluating the abdomen [4]. In supradiaphragmatic Hodgkin's lymphoma staging laparotomy has been performed for years to detect lymphoma manifestations in liver and spleen. Due to frequent perioperative and postoperative complications this procedure has recently been abandoned by the German Hodgkin's Disease Study Group although subdiaphragmatic manifestations may probably be missed in about 20% of the patients. Even using prophylactic spleen radiation the expected relapse rate will be 5% higher than previously [5]. As a non-invasive method PET might replace staging laparotomy and demonstrate involvement of additional abdominal sites.

Table 1. Staging procedures in malignant lymphoma

Basic	Special
Pathohistological documentation	Ultrasonography of the abdomen
Clinical examination	Bone scintigraphy
Routine laboratory screening	Endoscopy
Chest radiography	Gallium scintigraphy
CT of the abdomen	CT of the chest
CT of the pelvis	Cranial CT or MRI
Bone marrow biopsy	Liver biopsy
	Lumbar puncture
	Laparatomy

As a consequence of improved resolution of CT and MRI residual masses are more frequently seen after therapy. They are potential sites of lymphoma persistence or recurrence. In case of viable tumor, there are different ways to intensify treatment for example by means of autologous bone marrow transplantation. A large number of tests have been evaluated to diagnose relapse including erythrocyte sedimentation rate, MRI, and Gallium-scintigraphy [6]. Even for MRI the sensitivity was only 45% which is obviously too low to cope with the demands of oncology. Recently Newman [7] published a study of 16 patients using CT and PET for staging or restaging. PET localized 54 foci in 13 patients while CT showed 49. If PET proves to be more sensitive than routine procedures, this would be relevant for therapy.

Colorectal Carcinoma

The incidence of colorectal cancer is 50/100,000/year, figures of the frequency of local relapse vary between 9 and 20% [8]. Local recurrencies are mainly detected within the first thirty months after surgery. Only half of them can be operated with curative intent [9]. Those treated by surgery have a better survival than non-resected recurrencies. Therefore early detection is crucial. Current screening methods comprise physical examination including digital rectal examination, proctosigmoidoscopy (for rectal tumors), tests for faecal occult blood, and measurement of CEA serum levels [10]. Additional procedures like ultrasound or CT are only used in case of doubtful results e.g. elevated CEA. If the findings are still inconclusive, CT-guided biopsy, MRI, radioimmunoscintigraphy, and finally explorative laparotomy may be employed. In pilot studies, PET has been shown to be highly sensitive as well as specific for the detection of tumor relapse [11]. Should PET be able to differentiate ambiguous findings, some of the above mentioned methods might become unnecessary, and laparotomies could be confined to patients with localized tumor recurrence.

Lung Cancer

Lung cancer accounts for about 25% of all malignancies with an incidence of 60/100,000/year [1]. Early stages become apparent mainly as solitary pulmonary nodules, however, there are a lot of benign pulmonary nodules, too. Since the overall incidence is increasing with age, the probability of detecting cancer is higher in older than in younger patients. Sputum cytology is often not very helpful, because findings are positive only in about 15-20% of the peripheral lesions [12]. The results are slightly better though still unsatisfactory in patients with central lesions (sensitivity: 40-60%). Other current diagnostic procedures include CT, MRI, bronchoscopy with biopsy, and transthoracic needle biopsy. Only 90% of the biopsies are technically adequate and the reported sensitivity is 70-80% [13-15]. Radiological methods are hampered by low specificity. One of the best methods for characterizing ambiguous lesions is phantom-CT. It allows identification of benign nodes in 35-55%, which is still not satisfactory for clinical demands [16]. Thus, until now the only reliable way to diagnose solitary pulmonary nodules has been thoracotomy. PET has been reported to identify malignant lesions with a sensitivity of 83-95% and a specificity of 90-95% [17,18].

In bronchogenic carcinoma, metastatic spread to subcarinal lymph nodes indicates unresectable disease [19]. Although CT has proven to be more sensitive than plain tomography or chest radiography for detection of hilar and mediastinal adenopathy, it is not reliable enough to replace histopathological staging. Enlarged lymph nodes may be disease-free while normal sized lymphnodes may be involved with cancer. Careful nodal sampling at the time of mediastinoscopy or thoracotomy is therefore essential for accurate diagnosis [19]. Unfortunately sampling of subcarinal lymph nodes by mediastinoscopy is sometimes difficult and may lead to false negative results. With regard to overall evaluation of local or regional tumor spread CT and MRI provide similar information [20]. Correct preoperative staging is achieved in about 70% of the patients. In 5-10% thoracotomy reveals understaging which means that these patients are not curable by surgery [21]. Accurate prediction of subcarinal lymphnode involvement would therefore spare unnecessary operations. Treatment control in lung cancer is important although not crucial. Patient survival is usually limited by distant metastases, since no effective systemic treatment has been available until now [22]. Demonstration of residual masses has therefore no advantages and seems to be unnecessary in lung cancer.

Germ Cell Tumors

Germ cell tumors are relatively rare with an incidence of 5-8/100,000 males per year [1]. Depending on the stage of disease in 20-50% of those undergoing induction chemotherapy significant residual radiographic abnormalities will be present [23]. These patients are usually transferred to surgery. In earlier reports, about 40% of the resected masses revealed teratoma, 40% fibrous necrotic debris, and 20% viable tumor (Table 2, [24-27]). In recent studies more necrosis and less viable tumor was found in the postchemotherapy specimens. If we had a technique to identify residual viable tumor accurately, surgery would become unnecessary in two thirds of the patients.

Table 2. Pathohistological findings in residual masses of germ cell cancer

Author		Year	Patients		Necrosis		Teratoma		Viable tumor	
			n	%	n	%	n	%	n	%
Einhorn	(24)	1989	107	100	93	87	14	13	0	0
Sagalowski	(26)	1990	15	100	5	33	5	33	5	33
Rosenthal	(25)	1991	13	100	3	23	9	69	1	8
Fossa	(27)	1992	78	100	51	65	22	28	5	7
Total			213	100	152	71	50	24	11	5

Breast Cancer

In industrialized countries breast cancer accounts for 30% of all malignant tumors in women. The incidence is 60/100,000 females per year in Europe [28]. The number of breast nodules presented to physicians is twice as high. In the British Columbia Mammography Program abnormal results occurred in 9% of all examinations, but only 2% represented cancer [29]. These results are consistent with former studies. The current methods of clinical examination and mammography are highly sensitive but not specific, and therefore only useful for screening. In case of a suspect node, fine needle aspiration cytology will be obtained which has a high sensitivity and specificity but is technically inadequate in about 10% [30-33]. This rate will be lower if the puncture is performed by experienced investigators. PET might have the potential to be even more predictive as shown by a small pilot study (Table 3, [34]).

After diagnosing breast cancer, prognostic factors are needed to identify subgroups which do not need adjuvant therapy. Patient outcome is known to be significantly related to the extent of axillary lymph node metastases. On the other hand survival of patients with micrometastases measuring 2 mm or less is not significantly worse compared to patients without nodal involvement [36]. Since lymphadenectomy is exclusively performed for pathological staging but not for therapeutic purposes, non-invasive procedures are desirable to exclude lymphnode metastases larger than 2 mm in diameter. Whole body PET might be able to replace the different conventional techniques presently used for staging [36].

Table 3. Evaluation of suspect mammographic findings or palpable breast nodules with fine needle aspiration cytology (FNAC) or PET

Author		Year	Method	Pts.	Sensitivity (%)	Specificity (%)
Massod[a]	(30)	1990	FNAC	100	85	100
Zarbo[b]	(31)	1991	FNAC	13066	97	97
Vetrani	(33)	1992	FNAC	1153	93	92
Rotten[c]	(32)	1993	FNAC	1142	92	85
Adler	(34)	1993	PET	35	96	100

[a] 91% of all patients evaluable
[b] 82% of all patients evaluable
[c] 87% of all patients evaluable

Melanoma

Melanomas are estimated to account for 1.5-2% of all malignant tumors in Germany with an incidence of 10-15/100,000/year [37]. In case of an early stage without metastatic spread the 5-year survival rate is 75-80% [38]. The only curative treatment option is surgery. Patients with thin melanomas (smaller than 0.76 mm without evidence of regression) rarely have lymph node metastases while patients with larger tumors have a higher risk of harbouring occult metastatic disease. To date regional lymph node dissection is the only accurate staging procedure. Since only 20% of the melanomas in clinical stage I have micrometastases and need therefore to be treated by lymphadenectomy [39], it would be important to identify them and spare the majority of patients from useless operations. Preliminary results show a possible role of whole body PET for staging of melanomas [40].

Pancreatic Cancer

Pancreatic cancer has an incidence of 5-10/100,000/year [1]. Neither ultrasonography nor CT or MRI appear to be useful for the detection of small tumors [41]. The most sensitive method for pancreatic evaluation is endoscopic retrograde cholangiopancreaticography with an accuracy of 85-90% if technically feasible [42]. Endoscopic ultrasonography might improve the sensitivity for small lesions, the problem of reliable differentiation between focal chronic pancreatitis and malignancy, however, is still unsolved [43]. First results indicate that PET could be able to achieve discrimination [44].

Prostate Cancer

Prostate cancer is one of the two most common malignancies in men with an estimated incidence of 75/100,000 males per year [1]. Complete prostatectomy is a potentially curative procedure provided no metastases are present [45]. The results of CT and MRI in lymphnode staging are poor (CT: sensitivity 7%, specificity 96%; MRI: sensitivity 50%, specificity 100% [46]). Therefore pelvic laparoscopic lymphadenectomy routinely preceedes prostatectomy [47]. A non-invasive technique to replace this time-consuming procedure would be highly relevant. PET has been shown in other tumors to be sensitive for lymph node metastases, however, data for prostate cancer are missing.

Conclusion

Many diagnostic problems in oncology are still unsolved. There is an urgent need for additional methods which provide high accuracy in early tumor detection, staging or restaging, and localization of recurrencies. The results so far demonstrate the feasibility and clinical potential of PET. As shown above, it may be even cost-effective compared to routine staging procedures. If these encouraging results can be substantiated in larger trials, PET may play an increasing role in the management of oncological patients.

References

1. Boring CC, Squires TS, Tong T. Cancer Statistics, 1993. Cancer J Clin 1993;43:7-26.
2. Freedman AS, Nadler LM. Non-Hodgkin's Lymphomas. In: Holland JF, Frei E III, Bast RC, Kufe DW, Morton DL, Wechselbaum RR, editors. Cancer Medicine. Philadelphia, London: Lea and Felbinger, 1993: 2028-68.
3. Takvorian T, Canellos G. Hodgkin's Disease. In: Holland JF, Frei E III, Bast RC, Kufe DW, Morton DL, Wechselbaum RR, editors. Cancer Medicine. Philadelphia, London: Lea and Felbinger, 1993: 1998-2027.
4. Sandrock D, Lastoria S, Magrath IT, et al. The role of gallium-67 tumour scintigraphy in patients with small, non cleaved cell lymphoma. Eur J Nucl Med 1993;20:119-22.
5. Diehl V. HD-7 Protokoll der Deutschen Hodgkin Studiengruppe. Köln: Universitäts- klinik Köln, 1994:23.
6. Hill M, Cunningham D, Macvivar D, et al. Role of magnetic resonance imaging in pre- dicting relapse in residual masses after treatment of lymphoma. J Clin Oncol 1993;11: 2273-78.
7. Newman JS, Francis IR, Kaminski MS, et al. Imaging of lymphoma with PET with 2- (F-18)-Fluoro-2-deoxy-D-glucose: Correlation with CT. Radiology 1994;190:111-16.
8. Blijham GH. Kolorektales Karzinom. In: Seeber S, Schütte J, editors. Therapiekonzepte Onkologie. Berlin, Heidelberg, New York: Springer-Verlag, 1993: 191-200.
9. Minton JP, Hoehne JL, Gerber DM, et al. Results of a 400-patients carcinoembryogenic antigen second-look colorectal cancer study. Cancer 1985;55:1285-90.
10. Fantini GA, DeCosse JJ. Surveillance strategies after resection of carcinoma of thecolon and rectum. Surg Gynecol Obstet 1990;171:267-73.
11. Strauss LG. Application of positron emission tomography in colorectal carcinoma.Onkologie 1993;16:232-44.
12. Midthum DE, Swensen SJ, Jett JR. Clinical strategies for solitary pulmonary nodule.Ann Rev Med 1992;43:195-208.
13. Levine MS, Weiss JD, Harrell JH, et al. Transthoracic needle aspiration biopsy follow-ing negative fiberoptic bronchoscopy in solitary pulmonary nodules. Chest 1988; 93: 1152-55.

14. Khouri NF, Stitik FP, Erozan YS, et al. Transthoracic needle biopsy of the benign and malignant lung lesions. Am J Roentgenol 1985;144:281-88.
15. Utz JP, Patel AM, Edell ES. The role of transcarinal needle aspiration in the staging of bronchogenic carcinoma. Chest 1993;104:1012-1016.
16. Swensen SJ, Harms GF, Morin RL, Myers JL. CT evaluation of solitary pulmonarynodules: Value of 185-H Reference phantom. Am J Roentgenol 1991;156:925-29.
17. Kubota K, Matsuzawa TM, Fujiwara T, et al. Differential diagnosis of lung tumor with positron emission tomography: A prospective study. J Nucl Med 1990;31:1927-33.
18. Dewan NA, Gupta NC, Redepenning LS, et al. Diagnostic efficacy of PET-FDG imaging in solitary pulmonary nodules. Potential role in evaluation and management. Chest 1993;104:997-1002.
19. McLoud TM, Bourgouin PM, Greenberg RW, et al. Bronchogenic carcinoma: Analy-sis of staging in the mediastinum with CT by correlative lymph node mapping andsampling. Radiology 1992;182:319-23.
20. Rubin E, Sanders C, Harvey JC, et al. Diagnostic imaging and staging of primary lungcancer. Semin Surg Oncol 1993;9:85-91.
21. Bülzebruck H, Bopp R, Drings P, et al. New aspects in the staging of lung cancer. Cancer 1992;70:1102-10.
22. Perez CA, Pajak TF, Rubin P, et al. Long-term observations of the pattern of failureon patients with unresectable non-oat cell carcinoma of the lung treated with definiteradiotherapy. Cancer 1987;59:1874-81.
23. Roth BJ, Nichols CR, Einhorn LH. Neoplasms of the testis. In: Holland JF, Frei E III, Bast RC, Kufe DW, Morton DL, Wechselbaum RR, editors. Cancer Medicine. Phila-delphia, London: Lea and Felbinger, 1993: 1592-1619.
24. Einhorn LH, Williams SD, Loehrer PJ, et al. Evaluation of optimal duration of chemo-therapy in favorable-prognosis disseminated germ cell tumors: A Southeastern cancer study group protocoll. J Clin Oncol 1989;7:387-91.
25. Rosenthal MA, Stuart-Harris R, Tiver KW, et al. Single institutional experience with non-seminomatous germ cell tumours of the testis: local perspectives on a curable cancer. Aust NZ J Med 1991;21:857-62.
26. Sagalowski AI, Ewalt DH, Molberg K, Peters PC. Predictors of residual mass histo-logy after chemotherapy for advanced testis cancer. Urology 1990;35:537-42.
27 Fossa SD, Qvist H, Stenwig AE, et al. Is postchemotherapy surgery necessary inpatients with nonseminomatous testicular cancer and minimal residual tumor masses? J Clin Oncol 1992;10:569-73.
28. Miller AB. Causes of breast cancer and high risk groups. In: Harris JR, Hellman S, Henderson IC, Kinne DW, editors. Breast diseases. Philadelphia: Lippincott, 1991: 119-26.
29. Burhenne LJ, Hislop TG, Burhenne HJ. The British Columbia Mammography Scree-ning Program: Evaluation of the first 15 months. Am J Roentgenol 1992;158:45-9.
30. Massod S, Frykberg ER, McLellan GL, et al. Prospective evaluation of radiologically directed fine needle aspiration biopsy of nonpalpable breast lesions. Cancer 1990;66: 1480-87.
31. Zarbo RJ, Howanitz PJ, Bachner P. Interinstitutional comparison of performance in breast fine-needle aspiration cytology. A Q-probe quality indicator. Arch Pathol LabMed 1991;115:743-50.
32. Rotten D, Levaillant JM, Leridon H, et al. Ultrasonographically guided fine needle aspiration cytology and core needle biopsy in the diagnosis of breast tumors. Eur J Obstet Gynecol Reprod Biol 1993;49:175-86.

33. Vetrani A, Fulciniti F, Di-Benedetto G, et al. Fine needle biopsies of breast masses. An additional experience with 1153 cases (1985 to 1988) and a meta-analysis. Cancer 1992;69:736-40.
34. Adler LP, Crowe JP, Al-Kaisi NK, et al. Evaluation of breast masses and axillary lymph nodes with (F-18)2-Deoxy-2-fluoro-D-glucose PET. Radiology 1993;187:743-50.
35. Huvos A, Hutter V, Berg J. Significance of axillary macrometastases and micrometas- tases in mammary cancer. Ann Surg 1971;1:44-46.
36. Tse NY, Hoh CK, Hawkins RA, et al. The application of positron emission tomographic imaging with fluorodeoxyglucose to the evaluation of breast disease. Ann Surg 1992;216:27-34.
37. Garbe C, Orfanos CE. Epidemiology of malignant melanoma in Central Europe. Risk factors and prognostic predictors. Pigm Cell Res 1992;5:285-94.
38. Veronesi U, Cascinelli N, Adamus J, et al. Thin stage I primary cutaneous malignant melanoma. Comparison of excision with margins of 1 cm or 3 cm. N Engl J Med 1989;318:1159-62.
39. Balch CM, Milton GW, Cascinelli N, Sim HF. Elective lymph node dissection: pros and cons. In: Balch CM, Houghton AN, Milton GW, Sober AJ, Soong SJ, editors. Cutaneous melanoma. Philadelphia: Lippincott, 1992: 345-66.
40. Gritters LS, Francis IR, Zasadny KR, et al. Initial assessment of Positron Emission Tomography using 2-Fluorine-18-Fluor-Deoxy-D-Glucose in the imaging of malignant melanoma. J Nucl Med 1993;34:1420-27.
41. Brambs HJ, Claussen CD. Pancreatic and ampullary carcinoma. Ultrasound, computed tomography, magnetic resonance imaging and angiography. Endoscopy 1993; 25:58-68.
42. Pasanen PA, Partanen KP, Pikkarainen PH, et al. A comparison of ultrasound, computed tomography and endoscopic retrograde cholangiopancreatography in the diffe-rential diagnosis of benign and malignant jaundice and cholestasis. Eur J Surg 1993; 159:23-29.
43. Grimm H, Maydeo A, Soehendra N. Endoluminal ultrasound for the diagnosing and staging of pancreatic cancer. Baillieres Clin Gastroenterol 1990;4:869-88.
44. Bares R, Klever P, Hellwig D, et al. Pancreatic cancer detected by positron emission tomography with 18F-labelled deoxyglucose: method and first results. Nucl Med Comm 1993;14:596-601.
45. Paulson DF, Moul JW, Walther PJ, et al. Radical prostatectomy for clinical stage T1-2N0M0 prostatic adenocarcinoma: Long term results. J Urol 1990; 144:1180-84.
46. Hammerer P, Huland H. Zur Diagnostik des lokalisierten Prostatakarzinoms: Screening und präoperatives Staging. Urologe A. 1991;30:378-86.
47. Rioja-Sanz C, Blas-Marin M, Rioja-Sans L. Laparoscopic pelvic lymphadenectomy in the staging of prostate cancer. Eur Urol 1993;24:19-21.

5

ASSESSMENT OF GASTROINTESTINAL TUMORS WITH PET

Ludwig G. Strauss

Introduction

Therapy management of colorectal tumors poses several problems. One of them is the differentiation between recurrent tumor and scar lesions in the follow up after potentially curative surgery. Morphologic methods like computed tomography (CT) and magnetic resonance imaging (MRI) provide superior information about the size and location of a space occupying lesion, but are often not helpful in the classification of a mass. Positron emission tomography (PET) has been used for diagnosis of recurrent brain tumors since years [1-3]. Furthermore, DiChiro et al. showed that metabolic studies in brain tumors can be useful for noninvasive tumor grading [3]. Employing whole body positron emission tomographs, PET can be used for the diagnosis of recurrent tumors. By application of multiple radiopharmaceuticals information about perfusion and metabolism of recurrent tumors can be obtained. Furthermore, radiolabeled fluorouracil (FU) can be used to evaluate the kinetic and accumulation of this cytostatic agent prior to therapy.

Methods

A positron emission tomograph with two detector rings is in use at the German Cancer Research Center for patient studies. The system allows for the simultaneous acquisition of three slices with 8 and 11 mm slice thickness. Due to the use of 512 BGO/GSO detectors, a superior count rate performance at very low as well as high count rates is obtained as compared to the conventional block detector systems. Computed tomography (CT) is used in all patients immediately prior to PET to determine the target area for the following PET examination. PET measurements are performed for time intervals from 5 minutes (perfusion studies), one hour (FDG studies), up to 2 hours (radiolabeled cytostatic drugs). Cross sections are iteratively reconstructed using scatter and attenuation correction providing a spatial resolution of 5.1 mm in clinical use. The resulting slices allow for accurate measurement of tracer concentrations with an error of less than 3 % as compared to the true radiotracer concentration. Patlak analysis is performed to calculate regional metabolism if arterialized blood samples are available. Furthermore, in all patients a semiquantitative analysis of tracer accumulation is used in order to determine the uptake of a tracer in normal and malignant structures [4]:
SUV (standardized uptake value) = tissue concentration (MBq/g) / (injected dose (MBq) / body weight (g))

R. Bares and G. Lucignani (eds.) Clinical PET, 45–54.

Differential Diagnosis: Recurrent Tumor - Scar

Colorectal tumors belong to the most common tumors in oncology. In more than 30 % of all patients abdominoperineal resection of colorectal carcinoma is followed by local relapse within two years. Differentiation of recurrent tumor and scar presents a major problem in the management of these patients. Computed tomography (CT) does not permit reliable classification of soft tissue masses, as shown by Grabbe and Winkler, who reviewed the data of 51 patients with local tumor recurrence [5]. T1 and T2 sequences of magnetic resonance imaging (MRI) appear to be of limited value as demonstrated by Johnson et al. [6]. The accuracy of immunoscintigraphy (IS) is variable and dependent on the localization and size of the questionable lesion [7]. The diagnostic problems encountered evaluating possible tumor recurrencies suggest the application of PET, since this method can provide accurate, quantitative information about the metabolism of mass lesions.

FDG, one of the most common PET radiopharmaceuticals, was used in a study to differentiate tumor from scar on the base of local glucose metabolism in 43 patients. Since FDG is transported and phosphorylated like normal glucose but cellularly trapped thereafter, delayed images of FDG distribution reflect the local metabolic rate of glucose. Perfusion of the space-occupying lesions was evaluated with O-15 labeled water. Only patients with masses exceeding 1.5 cm in diameter were included in the study. Thirty patients had at least one biopsy suggestive for tumor recurrence, while thirteen patients had histologically proven scar lesions. Computed tomography preceeded PET

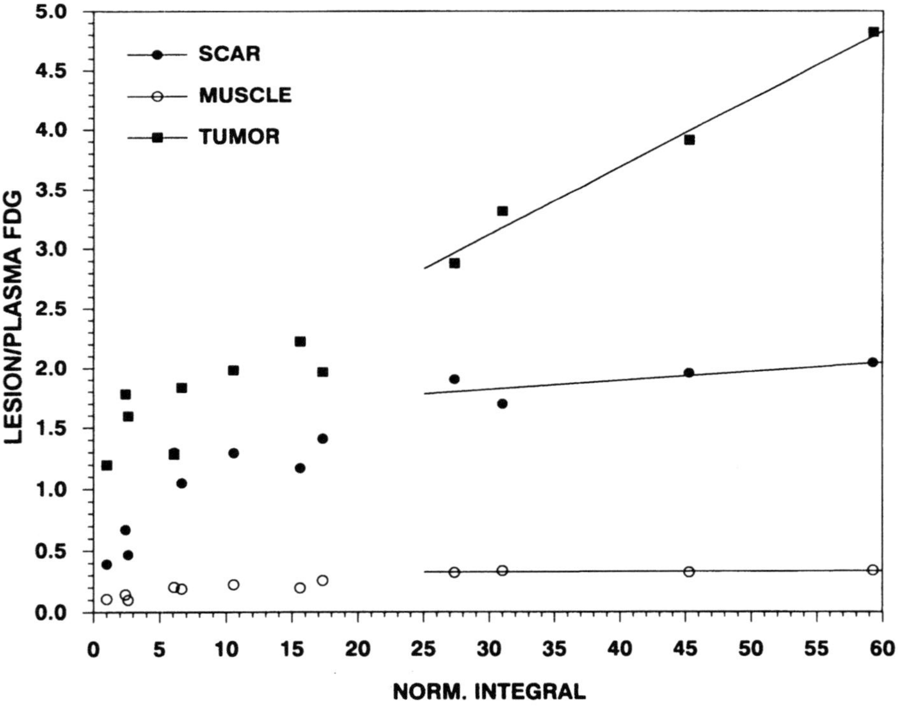

Fig. 1. Patlak analysis of tumor tissue and scar lesion

immediately to localize the lesion exactly. PET cross sections were iteratively reconstructed and scatter and attenuation corrected. Regions-of-interest (ROIs) were placed over the lesion as well as over the gluteal muscles, which served as normal reference. The tracer uptake was expressed as standardized uptake value (SUV).
All tumors were visible in the PET slices following intravenous FDG injection, while FDG uptake was low in scars. The Patlak analysis reflects the increased regional FDG metabolism in tumor tissue as compared to the scar lesion (Fig. 1). One hour after radiotracer application FDG uptake in malignant lesions was more than twice as high compared to normal soft tissue (Fig. 2). The quantitative evaluation of the FDG uptake demonstrates, that tumor and scar can be differentiated by one PET measurement one hour after tracer injection (Fig. 3). Only one tumor lesion was misclassified (Fig. 3). We noted a low correlation (r=0.67) between the intratumoral uptake of O-15 labeled water and FDG demonstrating that perfusion studies are not adequate for tumor differentiation. Information about tumor metabolism is required in order to classify doubtful masses.

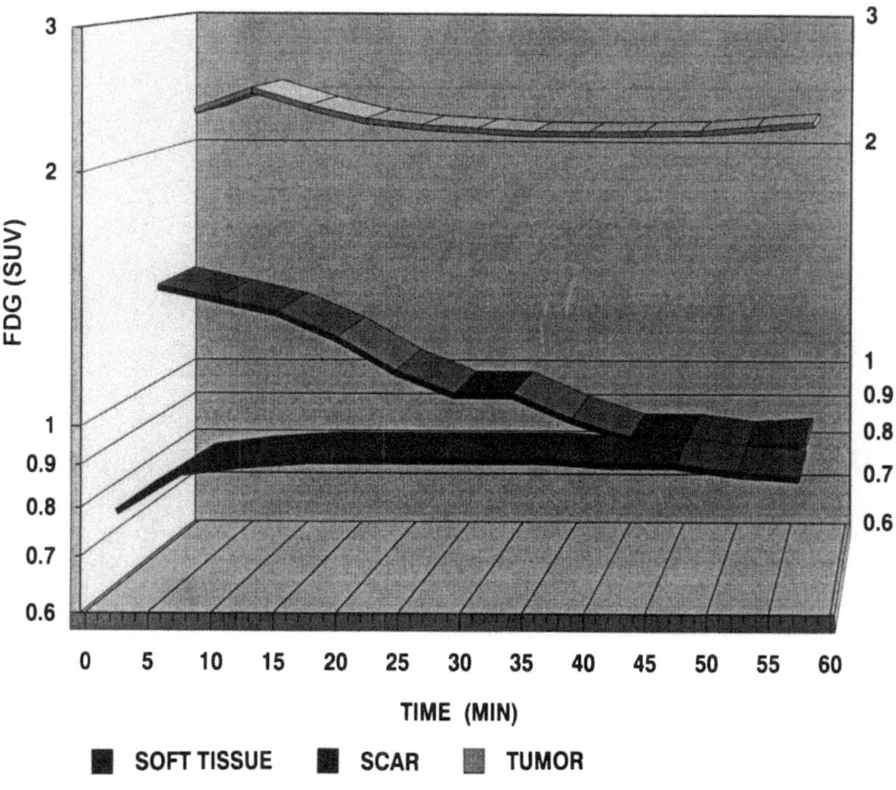

Fig. 2. One hour after radiotracer application FDG uptake in malignant lesions was more than twice as high compared to normal soft tissue

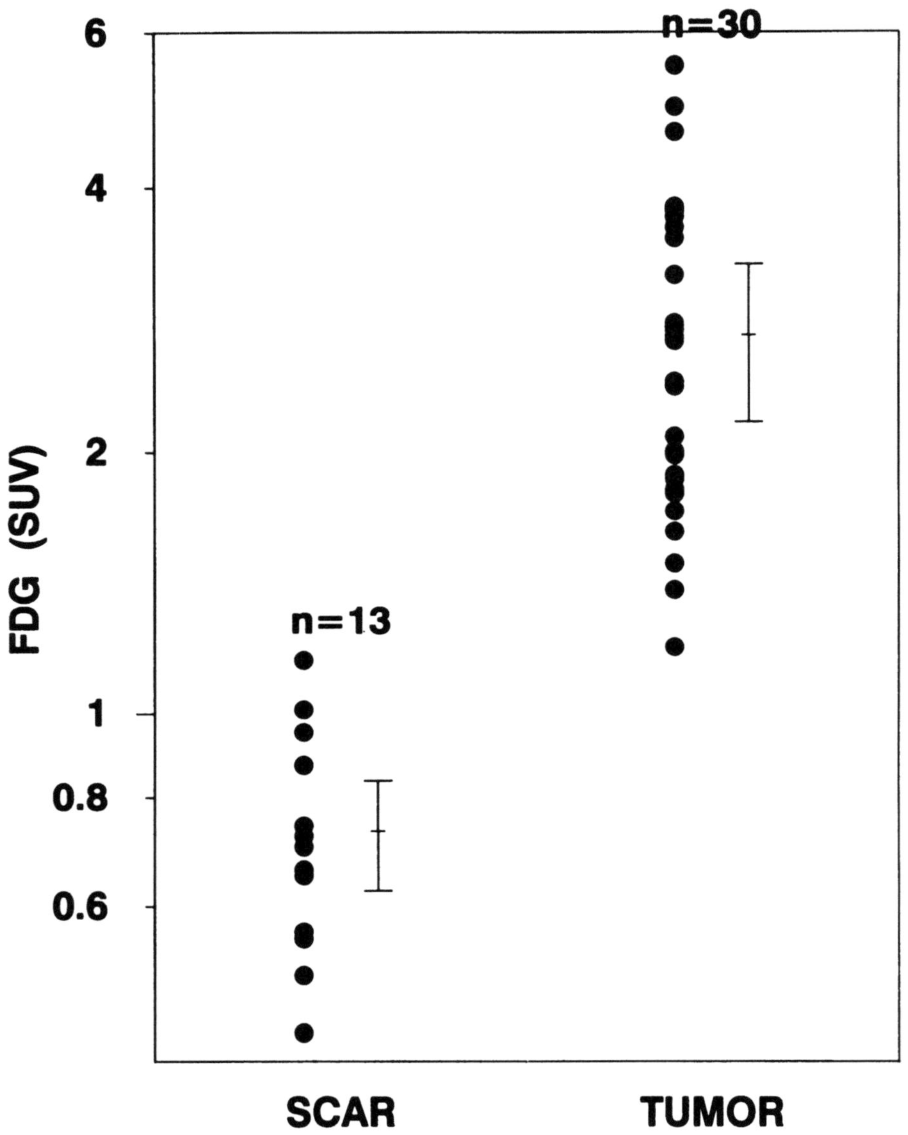

Fig. 3. The quantitative evaluation of the FDG uptake demonstrates, that tumor and scar can be differentiated by one PET measurement one hour after tracer injection.

Colorectal Tumors: Treatment of Hepatic Metastases

INTRAVENOUS CHEMOTHERAPY

Fluorouracil (FU) is the standard chemotherapeutic agent for treatment of hepatic metastases from colorectal cancer [8]. The metabolism of FU has been studied extensively in experimental studies. Tissue distribution studies, which analyzed the uptake of F-18 labeled pyrimidines in organs of AH109A tumor bearing rats, were reported by Abe et al. [9]. In 76 patients we used F-18 labeled FU in order to obtain kinetic data in metastases and the normal liver parenchyma. The standard treatment protocol includes the infusion of FU (500-1500 mg/m^2/24 h) for five days, followed by a three week interval without chemotherapy. To exclude potential effects of FU-infusions, PET was performed either preceeding the FU-therapy or at least one week following the last FU application in the drug-free interval. F-18 labeled FU (370-444 MBq) was injected together with 500 mg unlabeled FU during a short 12-minute period using an infusion pump. Images were acquired for 2 hours.
Visual analysis proved to be inadequate for evaluation of tracer uptake in metastases. Comparing tumor and liver background in most of the patients we failed to observe a clear difference in F-18 tumor concentrations in early as well as late images. In the aorta the highest F-18 concentration was noted after 10 minutes (Fig. 4), followed by a rapid

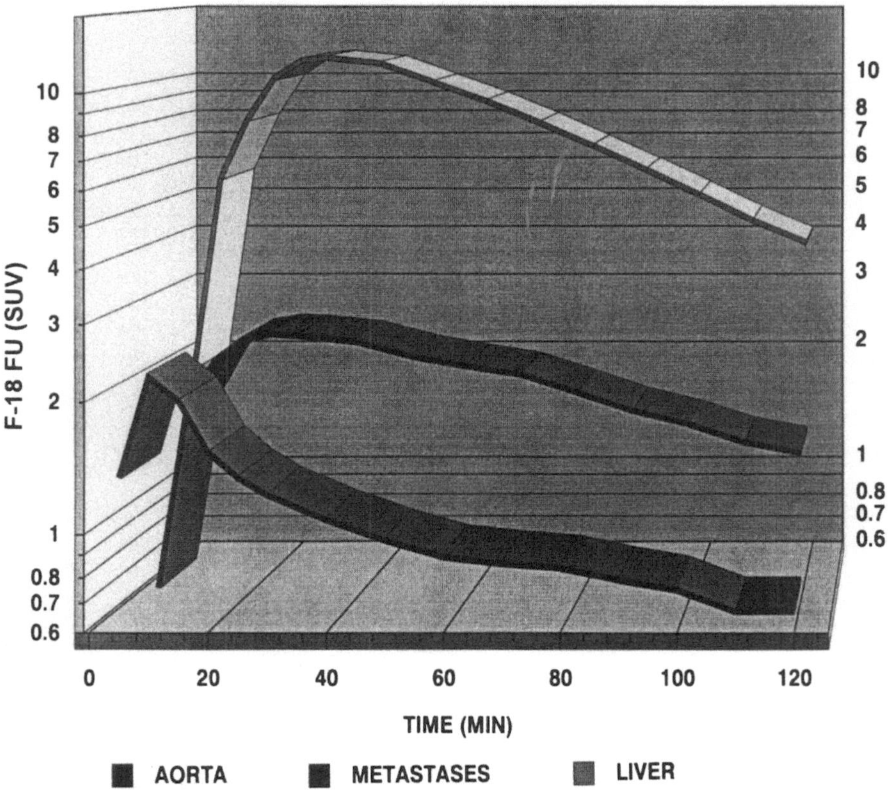

Fig. 4. Time-activity course of F-18 FU in the aorta, normal liver parenchyma and metastases.

decrease after the end of infusion. The maximum liver uptake was 11.4 SUV (mean value) with a standard deviation of 1.87 SUV. The time-to-maximum was 30 min (mean value), and ranged from 25-40 min after the onset of the infusion. The highest liver-to-aorta ratios were obtained 40-60 min after FU infusion. 5-FU uptake of individual metastases was low, and relatively constant after the initial distribution phase (Fig. 4). We found that the mean F-18 radioactivity in metastases was slightly less than one third of the concentration measured in normal liver parenchyma 120 min p.i. (Fig. 4). The tumor-to-aorta ratios were within 2-3 25-120 min after FU. PET images 8 min after FU infusion were evaluated to quantify FU transport into the tumor cells, while late images (two hours after injection of F-18 fluorouracil) were selected to estimate the metabolically active fraction of FU, since concentration of free FU in the plasma is low at that time. F-18 incorporation in metastases revealed considerable variation, as seen in the different time-activity concentration values (Fig. 4)

INTRAARTERIAL CHEMOTHERAPY

Regional application of FU has been used to improve the selectivity of drug uptake [10-11]. Theoretically, regional delivery can increase the drug concentration at tumor sites and lower systemic drug exposure when compared with systemic administration.

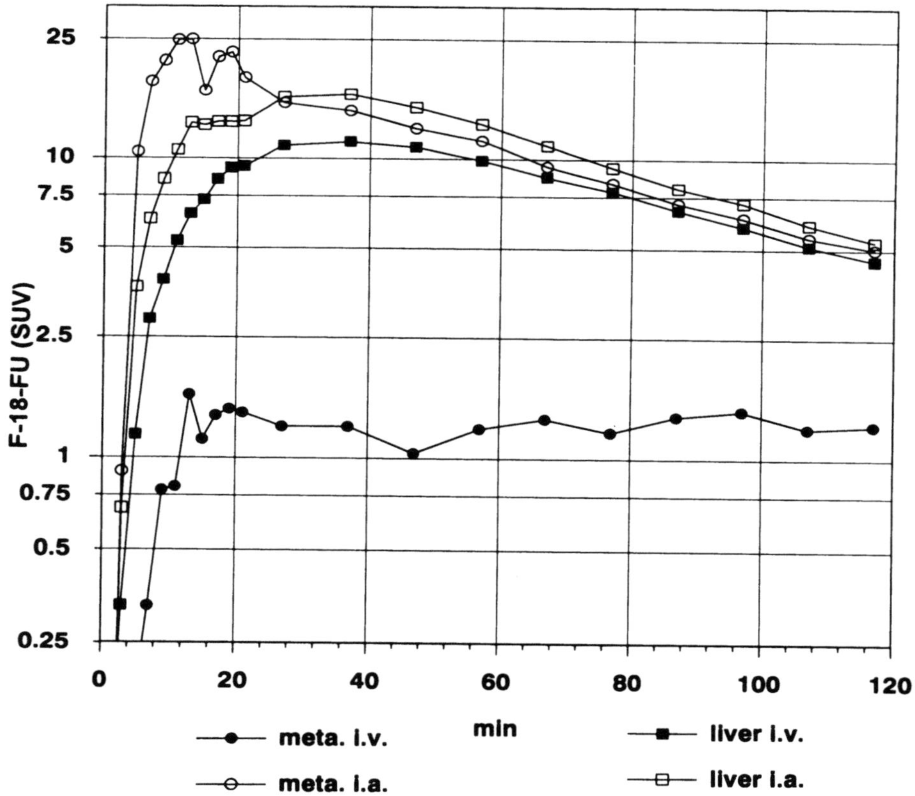

Fig. 5a. Time-course of F-18 activity following F-18FU administration intra-venously and intra-arterially in metastases and liver tissue.

We examined patients with F-18 labeled FU and O-15 labeled water to obtain quantitative data about perfusion and FU accumulation. Our primary goal was to evaluate the tracer concentrations following intravenous (i.v.) and intraarterial (i.a.) infusion of FU. Furthermore, we compared changes in perfusion and FU accumulation due to regional application.

We report on 26 examinations in 13 patients performed after intravenous as well as intraarterial tracer application. All patients had surgically implanted catheters in the gastroduodenal artery. Patients were examined prior to the first chemotherapeutic cycle or at least one week following the last FU application in the drug-free interval of the chemotherapeutic cycle. The results show that tumor perfusion (measured by O-15 labeled water) and early FU transport into the cells do not necessarily depend on each other. It should be noted that selective perfusion and increased FU transport with low FU elimination out of the cells are a prerequisite for an enhanced cytostatic effect of FU. Only a high FU accumulation, however, may lead to tumor regression.

While PET provides accurate information about changes of the F-18 concentration in tissue, no information is obtained about its biochemical nature. We tried to combine F-18-FU PET studies and F-19 magnetic resonance spectroscopy (MRS) following FU infusion in order to differentiate FU from its metabolites. Results of one patient are

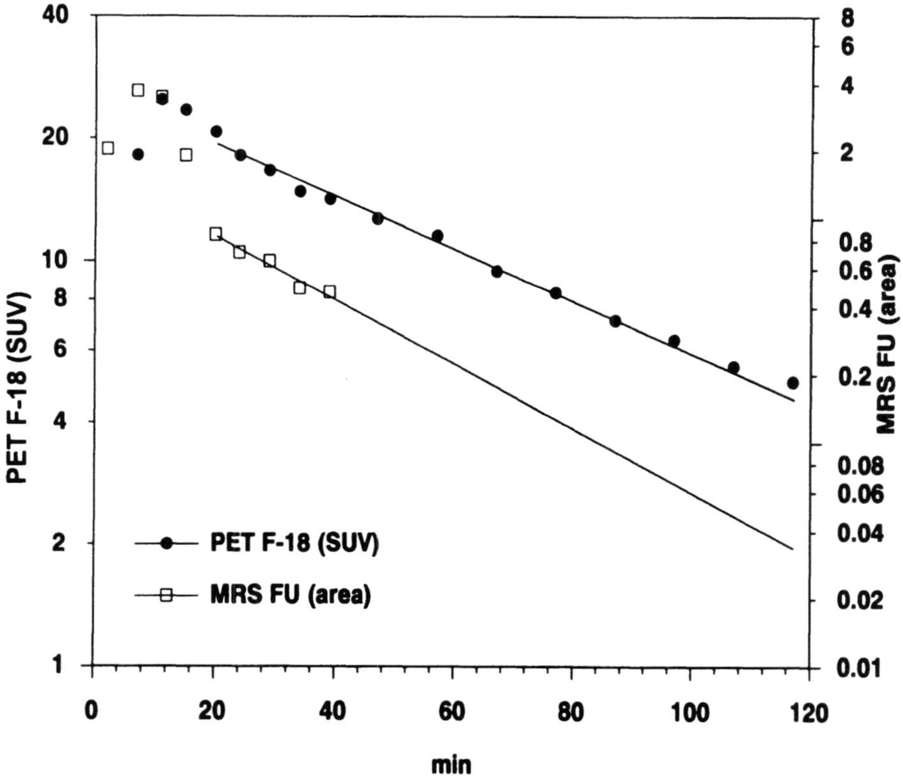

Fig. 5b. Time-course of FU assessed with PET and MRS.

demonstrated in Fig. 5a. The PET data after systemic infusion and regional application of F-18-FU show, that the regional approach increased the F-18-FU concentration values in the malignant lesion significantly (Fig. 5a). When compared with unmetabolized FU measured by MRS (Fig. 5b) regression functions of the data after the end of FU infusion demonstrate a comparable slope for both curves. Since MRS data represent the change in FU in the metastasis, we can conclude that F-18-concentration values measured by PET are likely to reflect the change in the intracellular FU concentration and do not represent FU metabolites.

FU ACCUMULATION AND TREATMENT RESULT

Hull et al. found no significant difference in the FU metabolite concentrations in plasma between responders and non-responders to FU chemotherapy [12]. They conclude, that detection of FU metabolites in tumor tissue is required for stating response to FU. Shani and Wolf showed in an animal study, that drug-responsive tumors had a 20:1 tumor-to-blood ratio 12 hrs post injection, while drug-resistant tumors had only a 4:1 ratio [13]. These data indicate, that measurements with F-18-FU in the tumor tissue may be helpful to predict response to FU chemotherapy in patients.

We examined patients prior to the first chemotherapeutic cycle with F-18 labeled FU and PET to obtain quantitative data about FU and its metabolites in metastases. Furthermore, CT studies were performed prior and after FU chemotherapy to calculate tumor volume from the cross sections. We compared F-18-FU concentrations obtained from PET images prior to chemotherapy with the tumor growth rate during chemotherapy. Our primary goal was to determine the correlation between these parameters in order to predict therapeutic outcome on the basis of PET.

We report on the evaluation of 22 liver metastases from 16 patients with colorectal carcinoma. All patients were examined prior to the first chemotherapeutic cycle. The standard therapeutic protocol included intravenous or intraarterial infusion of FU (500-1500 $mg/m^2/24$ h) for five days, followed by a three week interval without chemotherapy. Liver metastases were diagnosed prior to PET. Computed tomography immediately preceeded the PET examination, and was used to identify the region of greatest tumor diameter. The volume of each metastasis was calculated from CT cross sections using a three axis method (Volume = $(4/3)\cdot\pi\cdot a\cdot b\cdot c$). CT studies preceeded the first chemotherapeutic cycle and were repeated within 3-11 months after onset of chemotherapy. The growth rate was obtained from the volumetric data using the formula: growth rate = $\ln(Vol_2/Vol_1)$/(date of second CT study - date of first CT study), where Vol_1 was the volume of the metastasis prior to chemotherapy, and Vol_2 was the volume after chemotherapy. F-18 uptake was expressed as standardized uptake values (SUV). High FU accumulation was associated with tumor regression. We obtained a significant correlation coefficient for the tumor growth rate and the 2-h F-18-FU concentration (Fig. 6).

Chemotherapy with FU is still the standard treatment protocol for colorectal tumors. Depending on both the selection process and the response criteria used, the reported response rates have varied from 25 to 50 % [8]. Based on a literature survey, Köhne-Wömper et al. reported that the average response rate for hepatic metastases was 43 % in phase II studies using a continuous infusion of FU [8]. With moderate individual response rates, and highly variable population response rates, it is impossible to predict the individual response, or identify those who will most likely respond to therapy. Predicting response to FU therapy requires radiolabeling of the chemotherapeutic drug with the positron emitter F-18. F-18-fluorouracil is biochemically identical with the non-labeled cytostatic agent FU. Therefore, positron emission tomography with the F-18 labeled cytostatic agent FU. Therefore, positron emission tomography with the F-18 labeled drug provides the opportunity to determine the tissue concentration of FU. Interpretation of F-18 concentration values in a biochemical sense may be facilitated by compartment analysis. However, an input function for metastases is not easy to obtain. Therefore, we used MRS to measure the intracellular FU concentrations in metastases. The comparison of PET data of F-18-FU and MRS of FU in metastases demonstrates that the time-concentration values of PET after F-18-FU infusion mainly reflect the intracellular concentration of FU (Fig. 5b). These results are supported by Wolf et al., who evaluated the FU kinetic with F-19-MRS [14]. Since intratumoral FU is prerequisite for successful chemotherapy, the measurement of F-18-fluorouracil in metastases can help to identify those patients who meet this first criterion of therapeutic success. We were able to show, that the F-18-FU accumulation two hours after tracer infusion correlates with the tumor growth rate during chemotherapy (Fig. 6). Therefore, PET can be used to estimate the therapy outcome prior to the first chemotherapeutic cycle. Furthermore, different therapeutic protocols may be compared on the basis of F-18-FU uptake measurements. This noninvasive, quantitative evaluation of a cytostatic drug enables the oncologist to optimize and individualize treatment protocols.

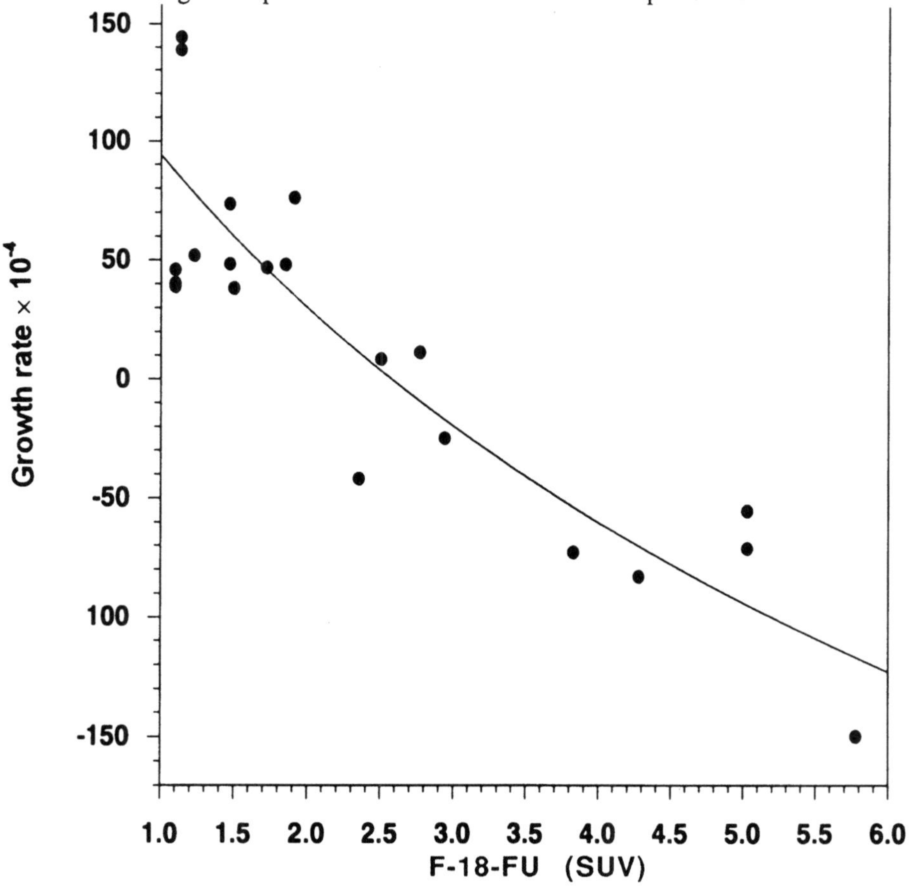

Fig. 6. Correlation of F-18FU accumulation and tumor growth rate during chemotherapy

References

1. DiChiro G, Oldsfield E, Bairamian D, Brooks RA, Patronas NJ, Mansi L, Kornblith PL, Smith BH, Sank VJ, Margolin RA: In vivo glucose utilization of tumors of the brain stem and spinal cord. In: Greitz T, Ingvar DH, Widen L, eds. Positron emission tomography. New York: Raven Press, 1985; 351-361.
2. DiChiro G: Positron emission tomography using [18F]fluorodeoxyglucose in brain tumors. A powerful diagnostic and prognostic tool. Invest Radiol 1986; 22: 360-371.
3. DiChiro G, Hatazawa J, Katz DA, Rizzoli HV, DeMichele DJ: Glucose utilization by intracranial meningiomas as an index of tumor aggressivity and probability of recurrence: a PET study. Radiology 1987; 164: 521-526.
4. Strauss LG, Conti PS: The applications of PET in clinical oncology. J Nucl Med 1991; 32: 623-648
5. Grabbe E, Winkler R: Local recurrence after sphincter-saving resection for rectal and rectosigmoid carcinoma: value of various diagnostic methods. Radiology 1985; 155: 305-310.
6. Johnson RJ, Jenkins JPR, Isherwood I, James D, Schofield PF: Quantitative magnetic resonance imaging in rectal carcinoma. Br J Radiol 1987; 60: 761-764.
7. Bischof-Delaloye A, Delaloye B, Buchegger F, Gilgien W, Studer A, Curchod S, Givel J-C, Mosimann F, Pettavel J, Mach J-P: Clinical value of immunoscintigraphy in colorectal carcinoma patients: a prospective study. J Nucl Med 1989; 30: 1646-1656.
8. Köhne-Wömper C-H, Schmoll HJ, Harstrick A, Rustum YM: Chemotherapeutic strategies in metastatic colorectal cancer: An overview of current clinical trials. Semin Oncol Suppl. 3, 1992; 19:105-125.
9. Abe Y, Fukuda H, Ishiwata K, Yoshioka S, Yamada K, Endo S, Kubota K, Sato T, Matsuzawa T, Takahashi T, Ido T: Studies on 18F-labeled pyrimidines. Tumor uptake of 18F-5-fluorouracil, 18F-5-fluorouridine, and 18F-fluorodeoxyuridine in animals. Eur J Nucl Med 1983; 8:258-261.
10. Strauss LG, Heim M, Jaschke W, Wetzel E, Schulze B, Beyer-Enke S, Georgi M: Intraarterielle Chemotherapie von kolorektalen Tumoren und Rezidiven. Tumor Diagnostik &Therapie 1986; 7: 225-230.
11. De Brauw LM, Marinelli A, van de Velde CJH, Hermans J, Tjaden UR, Erkelens C, de Bruijn EA: Pharmacological evalution of experimental isolated liver perfusion and hepatic artery infusion with 5-fluorouracil. Cancer Research 1991; 51:1694-1700.
12. Hull WE, Port RE, Herrmann R, Britsch B, Kunz W: Metabolites of 5-Fluorouracil in plasma and urine, as monitored by 19F nuclear magnetic resonance spectroscopy, for patients receiving chemotherapy with or without methotrexate pretreatment. Cancer Res 1988; 48: 1680-1688.
13. Shani J, Wolf W: A model for prediction of chemotherapy response to 5-fluorouracil based on the differential distribution of 5-[18F]Fluorouracil in sensitive versus resistant lymphocytic leukemia in mice. J Cancer Res 1977; 37: 2306-2308.
14. Wolf W, Presant CA, Kenneth LS, El-Tahtawy A, Albright MJ, Baker PB, Ring III R, Atkinson D, Ong R, King M, Singh M, Ray M, Wiseman C, Blayney D, Shani J. Tumor trapping of 5-fluorouracil: In vivo 19FNMR spectroscopic pharmacokinetics in tumor-bearing humans and rabbits. Proc Natl Acad Sci USA 1990; 87: 492-496.

6

POSITRON EMISSION TOMOGRAPHY IN DIAGNOSING LUNG TUMORS

Kazuo Kubota, Susumu Yamada, Masatoshi Ito, Kenji Yamada, Takehiko Fujiwara, Roko Kubota, Kiichi Ishiwata, Hiroshi Fukuda, Taiju Matsuzawa, Masao Tada, Tatsuo Ido

Introduction

Lung cancer is the leading cause of death in many countries. In Japan the mortality of stomach cancer has begun to decrease while that of lung cancer is still increasing (1991: 21% of all cancer deaths in male and 11.5% in female). The reasons for this situation are not only high incidence but also poor prognosis. Significant improvements are expected in all aspects of disease management: detection, diagnosis, staging, treatment, and treatment evaluation.
If chest X-ray or sputum cytology demonstrate findings suggestive for cancer, advanced imaging procedures like CT, MRI or nuclear medicine techniques are considered for differential diagnosis and staging. Since focal nodular structures as well as enlarged mediastinal lymphnodes may be frequently found after inflammatory or granulomatous lung disorders differentiation from malignant tumors has become a constant diagnostic challenge.

Computed Tomography

Due to superior spatial and contrast resolution computed tomography (CT) is more accurate than plain X-ray in evaluating nodules with regard to calcification which is an important sign of benign disease. Proto and Thomas [1] reported a 100% sensitivity, 54% specificity, and 79% accuracy in the differential diagnosis of solitary pulmonary nodules. However, the rate of inconclusive studies was as high as 21%. Density measured by CT cannot be regarded as absolute physical value but only as relative indicator of density depending from several variables. In order to standardize CT densitometry a specially designed reference phantom has been developed and was used in a multicentric study [2]. Application of this phantom and high resolution CT improved the detection of calcifications in lung nodules, however, 23% of the non-calcified nodules turned out to be false positive. In addition, 12 malignant nodules (7%) included calcifications, too. Furthermore tumor size and edge characteristics are suggestive but not reliable even if modern equipment is used [3, 4]. The results of four large CT studies [1-3, 5] are summarized in Table1. Only if CT reveals gross calcification, it is a reliable sign

R. Bares and G. Lucignani (eds.) Clinical PET, 55–66.

of benign disease (99%), otherwise findings are not histospecific.

Table 1. Differential diagnosis of malignant lung tumors by CT

Author		year	TP	FN	TN	FP
Proto	(Cincinnati)	1985	96	0	44	37
Zerhouni	(Multicenter)	1986	176	1	87	53
Siegelman	(Baltimore)	1986	283	0	176	103
Huston	(Rochester)	1989	26	1	32	53
total			581	2	339	246
			sensitivity: 99.7 %		specificity: 57.9 %	

abbreviations:
TP = true positive
FN = false negative
TN = true negative
FP = false positive

In staging of lung cancer, various size criteria have been used to define enlarged lymphnodes. In general, the sensitivity and specificity of CT to differentiate malignant from benign nodes depends on the diameter used for discrimination. Results ranging from 60-80 % in both sensitivity and specificity have been reported using either long axis or short axis diameters greater than 10 mm [6, 7]. Presence of tumor invasion in normal-sized lymphnode is a further cause of false negative results.

Single Photon Nuclear Medicine

Single photon nuclear medicine techniques to detect lung cancer have been reviewed recently [8]. ^{67}Ga scintigraphy does not appear to be useful for staging or differential diagnosis any more. ^{201}Tl imaging of brain, bone, and soft tissue tumors was considered to be promising, however, results in lung cancer are variable. Tonami [9] reported an accuracy of 76% for differential diagnosis of lung nodules using retention analysis and high resolution SPECT. Other groups have published worse results in both primary diagnosis and evaluation of mediastinal nodes. Specificity was reduced by ^{201}Tl uptake in benign lesions while high myocardial uptake compromized evaluation of the mediastine.

Positron Emission Tomography

Our first clinical study of lung tumors was done using [^{11}C]-L-Methionine [10]. Tumors were clearly visualized in eight lung cancer patients. Quantitative evaluation of Methionine (Met) uptake in tumor and normal tissue using differential uptake ratios (DUR) suggested that Met accumulation is closely related to tumor histology and the amount of viable or necrotic tissue determined by histopathology of resected specimens. However, because of the limited resolution of PET and retrospective type of this study it was difficult to evaluate the potential of PET for differential diagnosis. Therefore we started a prospective study comparing Met and [^{18}F]fluorodeoxyglucose (FDG) [11,12].

PATIENTS AND METHODS

Forty-six patients were examined by PET. They were referred to our hospital because of suspected tumors shown on chest X-ray films. The maximum tumor diameter varied from 0.5 to 6.0 cm. More than 60% (28/46) were 3 cm or smaller. PET studies were performed using either FDG or Met. Twenty-four patients were studied with Met (mean injection dose: 540 MBq), 22 patients with FDG (mean injected dose: 270 MBq). A PT931/04 PET scanner was used in 30 patients, an ECAT2 in 16 patients. Image analysis was based upon scans obtained from 40-50 min after injection. Regions of interest (ROI) were drawn around tumor (T) and muscle (M). The PET diagnosis was determined by T/M-ratios or visual interpretation. Afterwards the histopathological diagnosis was obtained and compared to the PET findings to calculate sensitivity, specificity, and accuracy.

RESULTS

The distribution of T/M ratios with Met was 5.3±2.0 (n=14) for malignant and 1.9±0.9 (n=10) for benign nodules ($p<0.001$) with a cutoff of 2.8. The T/M ratios for FDG were 4.4±2.2 (n=12), 1.5±0.2 (n=10) ($p<0.001$), and the cutoff = 2.0 respectively (Fig.1).

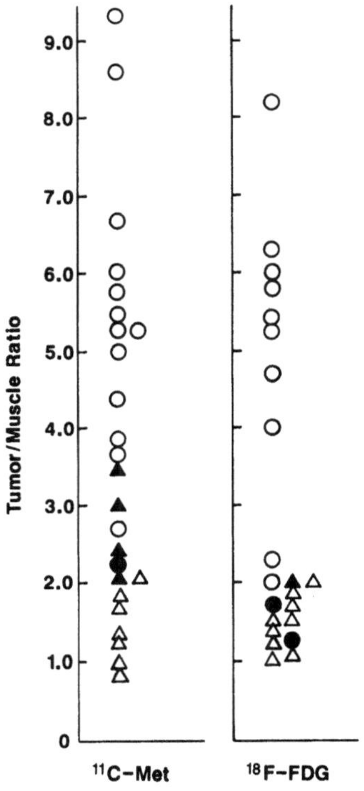

Tumor/Muscle Radioactivity Ratio by PET

Malignant
PET image
Positive Negative
○ ●

Benign
Positive Negative
▲ △

Figure 1. Tumor radioactivity of twenty-four patients studied by Methionine-PET and 22 patients studied by FDG-PET plotted as T/M ratio.A circle means malignant a triangle benign histopathology (from Ref. [12] with permission).

Most of the malignant tumors could be clearly differentiated from benign lesions using the T/M ratios mentioned above. However, some overlap produced false diagnoses. Tumors less than 1 cm in diameter seemed to be too small for accurate evaluation. For tumors larger than 1 cm the T/M ratios were separated into two groups of malignant and benign lesions suggesting that malignant tumors may have higher metabolic demands than benign tumors independent from tumor size. A typical PET image of lung cancer is shown in Figure 2.

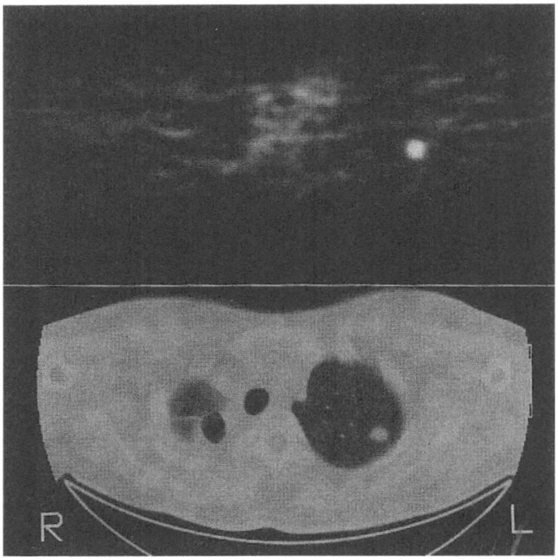

Figure 2. FDG-PET (45 minu-tes after injection) of a 1cm nodule located at the apex of the left lung.High uptake is present at the tumor site (adenocarcinoma confirmed by biopsy).

Using Met two granulomas, one aspergilloma, and one abscess were false positive. A 0.8 cm adenocarcinoma was false negative. The other 19 patients were correctly diagnosed. The calculated sensitivity, specificity, and accuracy of Met were 93% (13/14), 60% (6/10), and 79% (19/24) respectively. Using FDG a 0.5 cm squamous cell carcinoma and a liposarcoma were false negative. A granuloma was false positive. The other 19 patients were correctly classified. Thus, sensitivity, specificity, and accuracy of FDG-PET were 83% (10/12), 90% (9/10), and 86% (19/22). After the completion of this series, we investigated 17 futher patients using Met and 9 patients using FDG. So the final number of patients became 72, including 41 Met and 31 FDG studies. As final result Met showed a sensitivity, specificity, and accuracy of 90% (26/29), 67% (8/12), 83% (34/41), FDG revealed 89% (17/19), 92% (11/12), 90% (28/31) indicating that FDG is more suitable for differential diagnosis than Met.

DISCUSSION AND REVIEW

Studies from Europe [13, 14, 17] and USA [16, 18, 19, 20] yielded similar sensitivities (95-98%) and specificities (83-94%) than ours (Table 2). The Institute for Clinical PET recently published a retrospective survey of US PET-centers with a sensitivity and specificity of FDG-PET of 96% and 90% respectively [21]. Thus, more than 400 patients with lung tumors have been studied by FDG-PET in more than 10 PET centers in Europe, USA, and Japan. All agreed that PET imaging is accurate except for a few inflammatory lesions. Using Met similar results have been reported by Miyazawa [22].

They found that tumor uptake of Met correlated closely with the proliferation index measured by flow-cytometry.

Table 2. Differential diagnosis of lung tumors by FDG-PET

Author		year	TP	FN	TN	FP
Nolop	(London)	1987	12	0	0	0
Kubota	(Sendai)	1990	17	2	11	1
Strauss	(Heidelberg)	1991	86	1	10	3
Jacobs	(Dayton)	1992	17	0	8	1
Wahl	(Ann Arbor)	1992	5	2	4	0
Slosman	(Geneva)	1993	29	2	3	2
Pats	(Durham)	1993	47	1	16	1
Gupta	(Omaha)	1994	48	3	13	2
Hubner	(Knoxville)	1994	36	4	31	2
total			297	15	96	12
			sensitivity: 95.2%		specificity: 88.9%	

Several reports are also available dealing with the evaluation of mediastinal lymphnodes and staging. Knopp compared FDG-PET with histopathology and found FDG-PET to be more accurate than CT [23]. Wahl reported that mediastinal staging by PET was in agreement with surgery in 81% (22/27), CT only in 52% (14/27) of lung cancer patients [24]. The recent development of whole-body PET might open a new era in staging of lung cancer [25].

False positive FDG-accumulations have been published in tuberculosis, aspergillosis, and sarcoidosis [26]. Experimental studies using microautoradiography have demonstrated that there is a high accumulation of FDG not only in cancer cells but also in macrophages and young granulation tissue which may explain the mechanism of FDG uptake by inflammatory lesions [27]. An accurate method to avoid false positive findings still needs to be developed.

As for technical aspects, most groups did not calculate metabolic rates of glucose with arterial blood sampling. Semiquantitative parameters called DUR, SUV, or SUR (Differential or Dose or Standardized Uptake Ratio or Value: tumor radioactivity normalized by injected dose and body weight) are widely used and proved to be adequate except for obese patients. In the latter normalization for body surface [28] or by lean body weight [29] has been suggested. Uptake of FDG moreover depends on blood glucose levels. In patients with hyperglycemia tumor uptake of FDG drops significantly [30] which might cause false negative PET findings. Besides, DUR may vary widely with time [31]. In Met studies Met uptake by head and neck cancer is reported to decrease slightly after food ingestion [32]. Therefore PET studies with both FDG or Met should be performed under fasting conditions. In addition measurements of blood glucose, body weight,and height are recommended.

PET for Treatment Evaluation

Measurement of tumor size as demonstrated by plain X-ray or CT is regarded as standard method for treatment evaluation of cancer. However, radio- or chemotherapy induces tissue alterations such as fibrosis, necrosis, or lethal cell injuries creating the diagnostic problem that residual masses do not necessarily mean residual disease. There is an emerging need for methods able to monitor disease activity directly. Accurate evaluation of tumor viability would be beneficial for cancer patients. PET is expected to play an important role in non-invasive treatment control.

PRECLINICAL STUDIES

Tumor tissue responses to radiotherapy which can be measured by PET as has been shown experimentally. Using a rat tumor model, we calculated tumor volume, the amount of viable tissue within the tumor, and the tracer uptake after radiotherapy [33-36]. ^{3}H-thymidine and ^{14}C-methionine uptake showed a rapid and sensitive response to irradiation, preceded by both volumetric shrinkage and necrotic extension. Furthermore both tracers allowed to detect early foci of recurrence. FDG-accumulation was highly variable but steadily declining after irradiation. Changes were nearly parallel to the amount of necroses that preceded volumetric shrinkage and showed a linear correlation to the percentage of viable tissue. In contrast, thymidine (a marker of proliferation) underestimated the amount of viable tissue. Findings with Met were similar to those of thymidine (Fig.3). Our results suggested that thymidine as well as Met have the potential for rapid and sensitive monitoring of the effects of radiotherapy. Irradiation produces free radicals which induce injuries to enzymes, membranes, and DNA (Fig.4). Thus, reduction of thymidin or Met uptake reflects altered metabolism and cell death preceding cell autolysis observed in necroses. Reduction of tumor volume will not become apparent until a large proportion of the necrosis has been removed. We conclude that PET using Met demonstrates radiation effects immediately after irradiation and may thus beneficially influence management of patients undergoing radiotherapy.

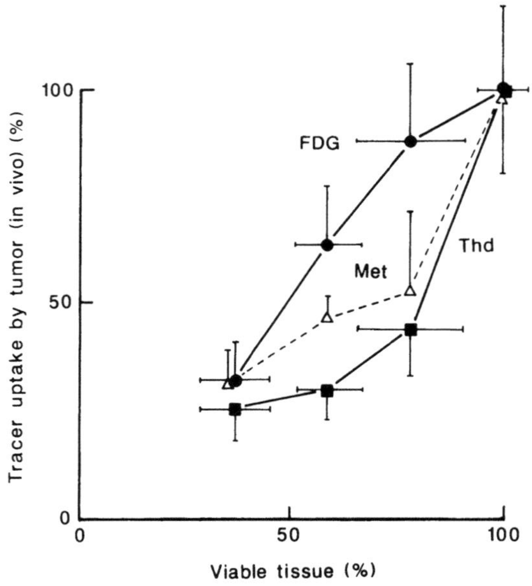

Figure 3. Tumor uptake of FDG, ^{14}C-Met and ^{3}H-Thymidine 1, 3 and 6 days after 20 Gy irradiation compared to quantitative histo-pathology of viable tumor tissue.The control data were assigned 100% (from Ref. [36] with permission).

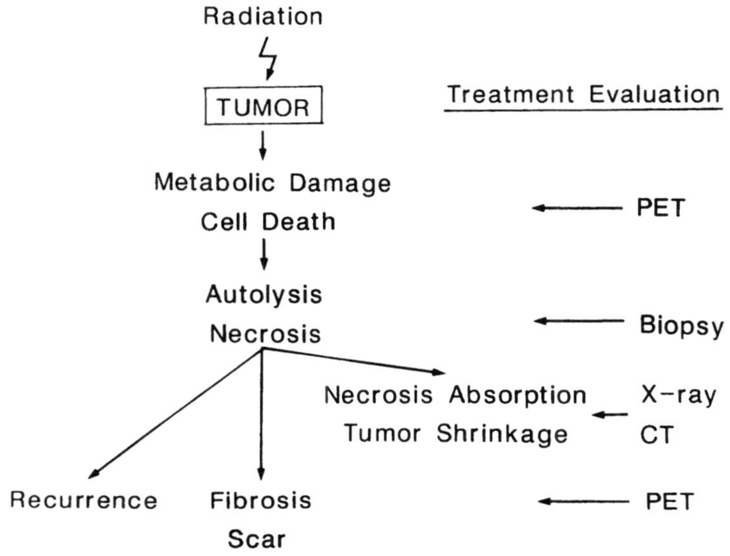

Figure 4. A hypothesis explaining the correlation of PET, CT, and histopathology in monitoring the tumor radiotherapy.

CLINICAL STUDIES WITH METHIONINE

We have performed long term follow-up studies comparing treatment monitoring by CT or PET in lung cancer [37]. In two patients the findings of PET were equal or superior to the evaluation of tumor volume measured by CT (Fig.5). Furthermore we compared early treatment effects on Met-uptake and tumor volume in order to predict the final outcome, e.g. recurrence or not [38]. Nineteen patients with lung cancer were studied. None had received any previous anti-neoplastic treatment. Two stage-1 patients had refused surgery, another stage-3 patient had received conventional radiotherapy of 50-70 Gy. None of the patients had active pneumonitis after radiotherapy at the time of PET and CT. Both were carried out before and within 2 weeks after completion of radiotherapy. The tumor uptake of Met was expressed as T/M-ratio, tumor volume was calculated by planimetry.

RESULTS

All patients revealed residual masses at the end of radiotherapy, and were classified according to the further clinical course (Fig.6). Ten patients (GroupA) showed no local recurrence or residual cancer. The Met uptake in this group significantly dropped after treatment as did the tumor volume. The reduction of Met uptake, however, was significantly larger than the reduction in volume. Five patients (Group B) had a local recurrence within 1 to 4 months after radiotherapy. They showed a smaller decrease of Met uptake as well as tumor volume compared to Group A. Four patients (Group C) had a tumor recurrence 11-18 months after radiotherapy. While tumor volume only slightly decreased the reduction of Met uptake was similar to Group A. All three groups had equivalent Met uptake prior to radiotherapy.

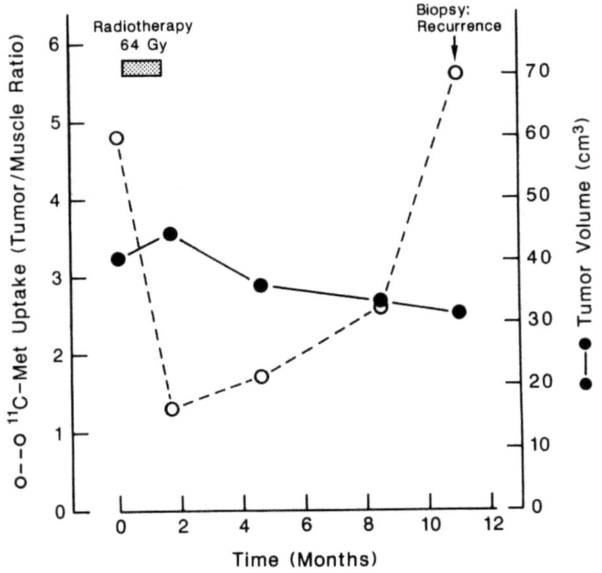

Figure 5. Tumor uptake of Met compared to tumor volume assessed by CT in a patient with large cell lung can-cer. Met-PET is more sensitive than CT to monitor responses to radiotherapy and recurrence (from Ref. [37] with permission).

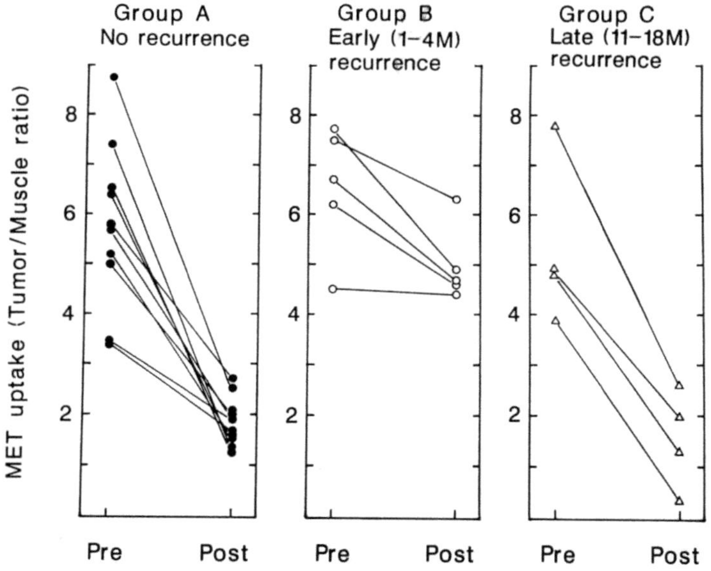

Figure 6. Changes in Met uptake pre- and postradiotherapy (from Ref. [38] with permission).

Using tumor volume as the only parameter we were able to differentiate the disease free (A) from both recurrence groups (B and C). However, we could not differentiate the early and late recurrence groups. In contrast, the latter groups could be clearly separated on the basis of Met uptake while no difference was observed between the disease free and late recurrence patients (A vs C), probably because the number of viable cancer cells at the end of radiotherapy was not large enough to be detected by PET. Using both parameters (reduction of Met uptake and tumor volume) a differentiation of the three groups became feasible. Thus, in case of residual masses demonstrated by CT, PET appears to be useful for evaluation of tumor viability.

DISCUSSION AND REVIEW

Using FDG Pats [39] and Kim [40] reported successful differentiation between recurrence of lung cancer and fibrosis. Both studies were performed more than 2 months after treatment and yielded a 99% sensitivity, 92% specificity, and 97% accuracy. However, different results have been published for monitoring radiotherapy by FDG-PET. False positive findings have been described in colon cancer [41]. Partial response as well as no response groups of lung or miscellaneous cancer patients revealed the same decrease in FDG uptake [42]. In addition FDG uptake within the radiation field has been reported to increase until 6 months after radiotherapy [43]. Therefore, one has to be very careful when interpreting increased FDG uptake after radiotherapy. Optimum timing should help to avoid interferences due to inflammatory reactions.
One of the main drawbacks of these studies is the small and heterogeneous patient population. Considering the costs and complexity of PET studies, in future multi-centric trials should be initiated, especially for topics related to cancer therapy. In our experimental studies, the intratumoral distribution of FDG and Met were clearly different. FDG accumulates not only in cancer cells but also in macrophages, fibroblasts, and granulation tissue [27]. In contrast Met is more selectively taken by cancer cells [44] and less affected by inflammatory reactions after radiotherapy [45]. This knowledge from basic research may be helpful for planning future clinical PET studies.

Conclusion

For the differential diagnosis and staging of lung cancer, PET with FDG or Met reveals high accuracy. PET is clearly superior to CT. It allows to avoid unnecessary surgery of benign lesions and to select the appropriate treatment modality. However, there are limitations in the detection of small lesions and due to false positive results in inflammatary disease. PET studies cannot replace pathohistology but may become relevant for the non-invasive diagnosis of cancer.
After treatment, CT may be altered by fibrosis, and biopsies are sometimes not easy to obtain. For the detection of recurrence, PET with FDG or Met revealed excellent results. However, increased FDG uptake may also be caused by post-radiotherapy inflammation. We need to know the optimal timing for PET to avoid interference by inflammatory reactions. PET using Met may be useful for early treatment evaluation, however, further studies to substantiate these findings are necessary.

Acknowledgements

We are grateful to Mr. Y. Sugawara for photography. This work was supported by grant-in-aid (04557047, 06454320) from the ministry of Education, Science and Culture, Japan.

References

1. Proto AV, Thomas SR. Pulmonary nodules studied by computed tomography. Radiology 1985; 156: 149-153.
2. Zerhouni EA, Stitik FP, Siegelman SS, et al. CT of the pulmonarynodule: a co-operative study. Radiology 1986; 160: 319-327.
3. Siegelman SS, KhouriNF, Leo FP, Fishman EK, Braverman RM, Zerhouni EA. Solitary pulmonary nodules: CT assessment. Radiology 1986; 160: 307-312.
4. Zwirewick CV, Vedal S, Millar RR, Mueller NL. Solitary pulmonary nodule: high resolution CT and radiologic pathologic correlation. Radiology 1991; 179: 469-476.
5. Huston J, Muhm JR. Solitary pulmonary nodules: evaluation with a CT reference phantom. Radiology 1989; 170: 653-656.
6. Staples CA, Mueller NL, Miller RR, Evans KG, Nelems B. Mediastinal nodes in bronchogenic carcinoma: comparison between CT and mediastinoscopy. Radiology 1988; 167: 367-372.
7. McLoud TC, Bourgouin PM, Greenberg RW et al. Bronchogenic carcinoma: analysis of staging in the mediastinum with CT by correlative lymphnode mapping and sampling. Radiology1992;182:319-323.
8. Abdel-Dayem HM, Scott A, Macapinlac H, Larson S. Tracer imaging in lung cancer. Eur J Nucl Med 1994; 21: 57-81.
9. Tonami N, Shuke N, Yokoyama K,et al. Thallium-201 single photon emission computed tomography in the evaluation of suspected lung cancer. J Nucl Med 1989; 30: 997-1004.
10. Kubota K, Matsuzawa T, Ito M, et al. Lung tumor imaging by positron emission tomography using C-11-L-methionine. J Nucl Med 1985; 26: 37-42.
11. Kubota K, Matsuzawa T, Fujiwara T, et al. Differential diagnosis of solitary pulmonary nodules with positron emission tomography. J Comput Assist Tomogr 1988; 12: 794-796.
12. Kubota K, Matsuzawa T, Fujiwara T, et al. Differential diagnosis of lung tumor with positron emission tomography: a prospective study. J Nucl Med 1990; 31: 1927-1933.
13. Nolop KB, Rhodes CG, Brudin LH, et al. Glucose utilization in vivo by human pulmonary neoplasms. Cancer 1987; 60: 2682-2689.
14. Strauss LG, Conti PS. The application of PET in clinical oncology. J Nucl Med 1991; 32: 623-648.
15. Jacobs MP, Mantil JC, Peterson CD, et al. FDG PET imaging of the chest. J Nucl Med 1992; 33: 975.
16. Wahl RL, Quint LE, Orringer M, Meyer CH. Staging non-small cell lung cancer in the mediastinum: comparison of FDG-PET, CT and hybrid anatometabolic fusion images with pathology. Radiology 1992; 185(p): 324.
17. Slosman DO, Spiliopoulos A, Couson F, et al. Satellite PET and lung cancer: a prospective study in surgical patients. Nucl Med Comm 1993; 14: 955-961.
18. Patz EF, Lowe VJ, Hoffman JM, et al. Focal pulmonary abnormalities: evaluation with F-18 fluorodeoxyglucose PET scanning. Radiology 1993; 188: 487-490.
19. Gupta N, Chandramouli B, Reeb S, Dewan N. Diagnostic evaluation of solitary pulmonary nodules. J Nucl Med 1994; 35: 76P, Radiology 1992; 184: 441-444, Chest 1993; 104: 997-1002.

20. Hubner KF, Smith GT, Raja S, Hunter K, Gould HR, Buonocore E. Positron emission tomography for evaluating chest masses. J Nucl Med 1994; 35: 220P.
21. Coleman RE, Cascade E, Gupta NC, Lawson M, Patz E, Rubin RJ. Clinical application and economic implications of PET in assessment of solitary pulmonary nodules: a retrospective study.1994 Institute for clinical PET, Fairfax VA, USA.
22. Miyazawa H, Arai T, Iio M, Hara T. PET imaging of non-small-cell lung carcinoma with carbon-11-methionine: relationship between radioactivity uptake and flow-cytometric parameters. J Nucl Med 1993; 34: 1886-1891.
23. Knopp MV, Strauss LG, Bischoff H, et al. Assessment of the potential clinical role of PET in the staging of thoracic adenopathy. Radiology 1991; 181P: 250.
24. Wahl RL, Quint LE, Greenough RL, Meyer CR, White RI, Orringer MB. Staging of mediastinal non-small cell lung cancer with FDG-PET, CT and fusion images: preliminary prospective evaluation. Radiology 1994; 191: 371-377.
25. Rege SD, Hoh CK, Glaspy JA, et al. Imaging of pulmonary mass lesions with whole-body positron emission tomography and fluorodeoxyglucose. Cancer 1993; 72: 82-90.
26. Lewis PJ and Salama A. Uptake of fluorine-18-fluorodeoxyglucose in sarcoidosis. J Nucl Med 1994; 35: 1647-1649.
27. Kubota R, Yamada S, Kubota K, Ishiwata K, Tamahashi N, Ido T. Intratumoral distribution of fluorine-18-fluorodeoxyglucose in vivo: high accumulation in macrophages and granulation tissues studied by microautoradiography. J Nucl Med 1992; 33: 1972-1980.
28. Kim CK, Gupta NC, Chandramouli B, Alavi A. Standardized uptake values of FDG: body surface area correction is preferable to body weight correction. J Nucl Med 1994; 35: 164-167.
29. Zasadny KR, Wahl RL. Standardized uptake values of normal tissues at PET with (fluorine-18)-fluoro-2-deoxy-D-glucose: variations with body weight and a method for correction. Radiology 1993; 189: 847-850.
30. Langen KJ, Braun U, Kops R, et al. The influence of plasma glucose levels on fluorine-18-fluorodeoxyglucose uptake in bronchial carcinomas. J Nucl Med 1993; 34: 355-359.
31. Hamberg LM, Hunter GJ, Alpert NM, Choi NC, Babich JW, Fischman AJ. The dose uptake ratio as an index of glucose metabolism: useful parameter or oversimplification? J Nucl Med 1994; 35: 1308-1312.
32. Lindholm P, Leskinen-Kallio S, Kirvela O, et al. Head and neck cancer: effect of food ingestion on uptake of C-11 methionine. Radiology 1994; 190: 863-867.
33. Kubota K, Matsuzawa T, Takahashi T, et al. Rapid and sensitive response of carbon-11-L-methionine tumor uptake to irradiation. J Nucl Med 1989; 30: 2012-2016.
34. Kubota K, Ishiwata K, Yamada S, et al. Dose-responsive effect of radiotherapy on the tumor uptake of L-methyl-11-C methionine; feasibility for monitoring recurrence of tumor. Nucl Med Biol 1992; 19: 27-32.
35. Kubota K, Ishiwata K, Kubota R, et al. Tracer feasibility for monitoring tumor radiotherapy: a quadruple tracer study with fluorine-18-fluorodeoxyglucose or fluorine-18-fluorodeoxyuridine, L-methyl-^{14}C methionine,6-^{3}H thymidine, and Gallium-67.J Nucl Med 1991; 32: 2118-2123.
36. Kubota K, Kubota R, Yamada S. FDG accumulation in tumor tissue (Editorial). J Nucl Med 1993; 34: 419-421.
37. Kubota K, Yamada S, Ishiwata K, Ito M, Ido T. Positron emission tomography for treatment evaluation and recurrence detection compared with CT in long-term follow-up cases of lung cancer. Clin Nucl Med 1992; 17: 877-881.
38. Kubota K, Yamada S, Ishiwata K, et al. Evaluation of the treatment response of lung cancer with positron emission tomography and L-methyl-^{11}C methionine:a preliminary study. Eur J Nucl Med 1993; 20: 495-501.
39. Patz EF, Lowe VJ, Hoffman JM, Paine SS, Harris LK, Goodman PC. Persistent or recurrent bronchogenic carcinoma: detection with PET and 2-(F-18)-2-Deoxy-D glucose. Radiology 1994; 191: 379-382.

40. Kim EE, Garcia JR, Wong FCL, et al. Differentiation of thoracic tumors from post-treatment changes using PET with F-18 FDG and C-11 Methionine. J Nucl Med 1994; 35: 76P.
41. Engenhart R, Kimmig BN, Strauss LG, et al. Therapy monitoring of presacral recurrences after high-dose irradiation: value of PET, CT, CEA and pain score. Strahlen-ther Onkol 1992; 168: 203-212.
42. Ichiya Y, Kuwabara Y, Otsuka M, et al. Assessment of response to cancer therapy using fluorine-18-fluorodeoxyglucose and positron emission tomography. J Nucl Med 1991; 32: 1655-1660.
43. Lowe VJ, Hebert ME, Hawk TC, Anscher MS, Coleman RE. Chestwall FDG accumulation in serial FDG-PET images in patients being treated for bronchogenic carcinoma. J Nucl Med 1994; 35: 76P.
44. Kubota R, Kubota K, Yamada S, et al. Methionine uptake by tumor tissue: a micro-autoradiographic comparison with FDG. J Nucl Med 1995.
45. Kubota K, Kubota R, Yamada S, Tada M. Effects of radiotherapy on the cellular uptake of carbon-14 labeled L-methionine in tumor tissue. Nucl Med Biol 1995.

7

ASSESSMENT OF HEMATOLOGICAL MALIGNANCIES WITH PET

Roland Bares

Hematological malignancies mainly comprise the various types of malignant lymphoma and multiple myeloma. While diagnosis of the latter is based on laboratory findings and bone marrow biopsy, the most important clinical sign of malignant lymphoma is lymphnode enlargement. Imaging procedures play therefore an important role for staging as well as treatment control. Plain x-ray techniques, computed tomography, and ultrasonography are all aiming at evaluation of lymphnode size assuming that lymphnode involvement is present if the diameter is exceeding 1.0 - 1.5cm [1,2]. However, even smaller lymphnodes may contain lymphoma infiltrations. On the other hand, lymphnode enlargement may also be due to inflammatory or granulomatous disease. Therefore sensitivity as well as specificity of morphologically based lymphnode evaluation is limited. The same is true for the assessment of liver or spleen and treatment control. While reduction of lymphoma size is generally accepted as sign of response, lymphoma persistence is difficult to interprete. Residual masses may contain viable lymphoma, necrotic tissue, or variable amounts of both. Until now definite differentiation can only be achieved by biopsy which inheres the possibility of sampling errors and serious side effects. Alternative non-invasive diagnostic approaches are therefore needed.

Scintigraphic Techniques

For more than two decades Gallium (^{67}Ga) scintigraphy has been used for staging and re-staging of malignant lymphoma [3]. After iv injection Gallium is predominantly bound to plasma transferrin and accumulates in lymphoma and other tumors expressing transferrin receptors. Clinical as well as experimental data show that uptake of ^{67}Ga indicates lymphoma viability and might therefore be suitable for assessment of residual masses [4,5,6,7]. Although there is some controversy about the results in different types of lymphoma, it can be stated that using adequate equipment and imaging techniques (high dose SPECT) sensitivities and specificities of 80% or more can be achieved [3]. Principal drawbacks, which have prevented general acceptance of this technique, are poor spatial resolution due to high energy gamma emission, long investigation periods (up to 14 days), and high radiation exposure (41 mSv/370 MBq compared to 6 mSv/300 MBq [^{18}F]Fluorodeoxyglucose (FDG) [8]).
Recently somatostatin receptor scintigraphy using ^{111}In labelled octreotide has been applied for lymphoma imaging, too [9,10]. Somatostatin receptors are present on more

R. Bares and G. Lucignani (eds.) Clinical PET, 67–74.

than 80% of Hodgkin as well as non-Hodgkin lymphomas and may therefore be used as target to detect lymphoma manifestations throughout the body [11]. Since activated lymphocytes are also receptor-positive, false positive findings may occur in benign conditions, e.g. inflammation, granuloma. False negative findings are mainly due to small size (<2cm in diameter) or localization in the abdomen (lesions are obscured by bowel radioactivity or superposition by liver or spleen). Since the reported sensitivity and specificity of somatostatin receptor scintigraphy is not superior to CT or FDG-PET [9], diagnostic relevance of this new technique is still subject of discussion.

Another potential tracer for malignant lymphoma is ^{201}Tl. Advantages compared to ^{67}Ga and ^{111}In octreotide are rapid accumulation and higher spatial resolution using low-energy gamma camera equipment. On the other hand, reliable evaluation of the abdomen is hampered by high bowel radioactivity so that clinical impact of this technique appears to be low [12]. Hexakis-2-methoxy-isobutylisonitrile (MIBI) labelled with ^{99m}Tc has been used for imaging of lymphoma, too. Based on experimental data demonstrating that MIBI might be useful to study presence of multidrug resistant P-glycoprotein [13], a pilot study was performed in a small number of untreated lymphoma patients. Results so far indicate that MIBI-uptake correlates with clinical response to chemotherapy [14]. Larger trials are needed to substantiate these data, in particular to analyze whether MIBI-scintigraphy may play a role for treatment selection. Table 1 gives a summary of the results of ^{67}Ga, ^{201}Tl, and octreotide scanning in malignant lymphoma.

Table 1. Results of different scintigraphic techniques in detecting malignant lymphoma.

Author		Year	Method	Pts.	Sensitivity (%)	Specificity (%)
Tumeh	[5]	1987	Gallium	40	94	100
Kostakoglu	[6]	1992	Gallium	30	96	80
Front	[7]	1993	Gallium	68	95	89
Sehweil	[12]	1989	Thallium	13	85	not available
Bares	[9]	1993	Octreotide	18	66	90
Lipp	[10]	1995	Octreotide	41	47	40

PET in Malignant Lymphoma

Several positron emitting radiopharmaceuticals have been used to image malignant lymphoma so far. Since increased glucose metabolism as metabolic sign of malignant disease has become widely accepted, [^{18}F]fluorodeoxyglucose (FDG) was chosen in most of the studies. Paul was the first to scan FDG in a small series of 5 untreated lymphoma patients using a conventional gamma camera [15]. Compared to ^{67}Ga scans FDG proved to be superior in detecting lymphoma manifestations. Furthermore repeated scans in a patient suffering from retroperitoneal sinus carcinoma indicated that FDG might be suitable to evaluate treatment effects. These results were confirmed by Okada who found positive correlations between FDG-uptake, the tumor/non-tumor ratio, glucose utilization rate and prognosis or proliferative activity of untreated malignant lymphoma [16,17]. Compared to ^{67}Ga-SPECT, contrast and image quality of FDG-PET was clearly superior. Leskinen-Kallio studied 14 patients with untreated non-Hodgkin lymphoma using FDG and ^{11}C labelled methionine [18]. While uptake as well as transport were higher for methionine, FDG appeared to be more suitable to differentiate high-grade from intermediate or low-grade lymphoma. Recently Schönberger [19] proposed whole body PET as initial staging procedure for untreated lymphoma. In 7 out of 17 patients PET identified previously unknown lesions causing up-grading in 4 of them. Similar results were reported by Hoh [20]. Thus, due to high FDG-uptake and contrast to surrounding normal tissue (Fig.1) sensitivity of PET in untreated lymphoma appears to be virtually 100%.

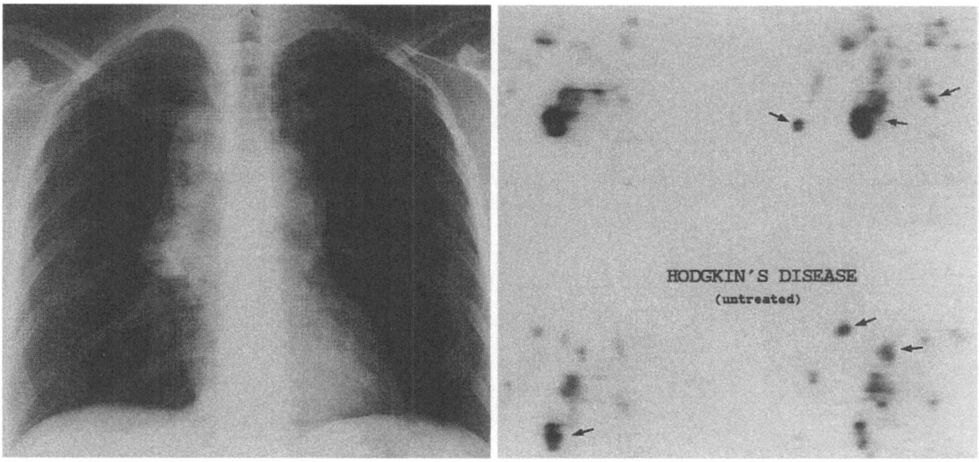

Figure 1. Plain thorax x-ray (left) and FDG-PET (right) of a 23 years old female patient with untreated Hodgkin's disease. Note intense FDG-accumulation in multiple lymphoma lesions (arrows).

FDG-PET studies were also performed to evaluate treatment effects. Newman correlated CT-findings in 16 patients with various types of lymphoma with PET [21]. While all sites with proven adenopathy were positive in PET, 3 patients with negative findings at subsequent staging laparatomy were negative. Our own group investigated 47 patients after completion of chemotherapy [22]. Visual analysis of static PET-scans allowed accurate differentiation of 26 residual masses shown by CT (accuracy: 96%; examples Figs. 2 and 3). Furthermore, unexpected hypermetabolic lesions were detected in 9 out of 21 patients classified as complete remission on the basis of CT (Table 2). A comparative study of Garcia [23] in 20 patients with treated bone lymphoma revealed that FDG-PET was superior to Gallium scanning, in particular with regard to specificity of positive findings (PET: 100%, ^{67}Ga: 67%). Planar FDG-scans might also be useful for treatment evaluation as shown by Hoekstra [24]. After effective chemotherapy FDG-uptake rapidly decreases as sign of response. Detection of small residual lesions, however, might be more difficult, since spatial resolution of conventional gamma cameras equipped with 511 keV collimators is poor. In general FDG-PET proved to be highly accurate in identifying viable lymphoma regardless of type and location.

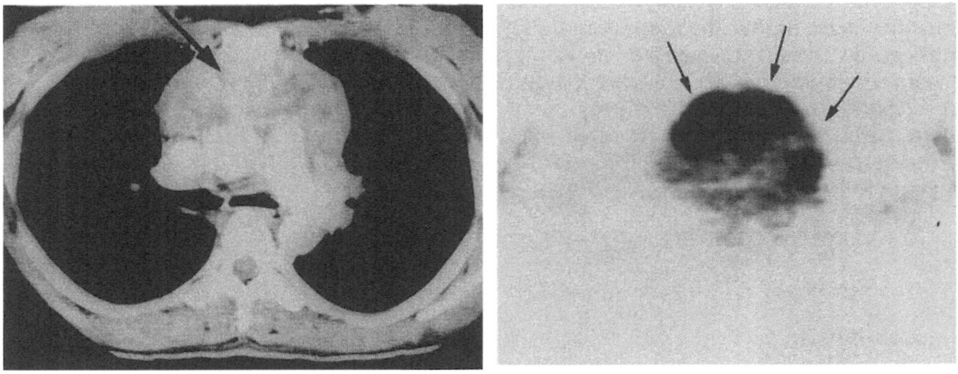

Figure 2. CT (left) and FDG-PET (right) in a 19 years old female with high-grade NHL pretreated by 4 course of polychemotherapy. Note high FDG-uptake in residual lymphoma masses indicating viable tumor (confirmed by biopsy).

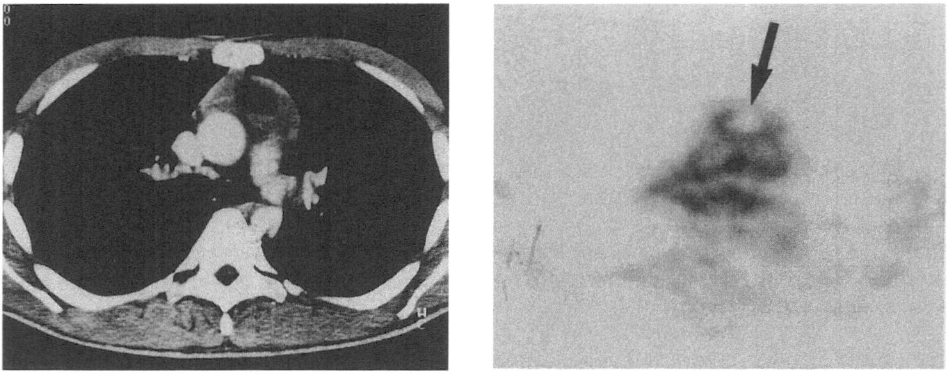

Figure 3. CT (left) and FDG-PET (right) in 22-years old male with residual mediastinal Hodgkin´s lymphoma. Absence of significant FDG-accumulation indicates necrosis confirmed by CT-guided biopsy and clinical course.

Table 2. Results of FDG-PET for treatment control after chemotherapy

Clinical Diagnosis	Residual Masses	Increased FDG-Uptake	
Partial Remission	26	16/26	(61.5%)
viable tissue[a]	17/26	16/17	(94.1%)
necrosis[a]	9/26	0/9	
Complete Remission	0/21	9/21	(42.8%)
recurrency[b]	0/7	7/7	(100%)
disease-free[b]	0/14	2/14	(14.3%)

[a] confirmed by biopsy [b] confirmed by clinical course (>6 months)

Besides FDG ^{11}C labelled methionine and thymidine have also been used for evaluation of malignant lymphoma. As mentioned above uptake of methionine was very high exceeding that of FDG when compared intraindividually [18]. Clinical usefulness, however, seems to be limited by the short physical half-life of ^{11}C making whole body surveys not feasible. The same is true for ^{11}C labelled thymidine which provides information about proliferation and (probably) individual prognoses non-invasively [25].

Clinical Implications

Three relevant diagnostic problems of malignant lymphoma might be solved by the use of FDG-PET:

1) as whole-body procedure PET should be able to detect disease in normal-sized lymphnodes (and eventually spleen) and might therefore modify (or even replace) staging by conventional methods.
2) since PET diagnoses active disease on the basis of metabolism not size, those patients with residual masses due to scar or necroses might be spared from further treatment.
3) clinical as well as experimental data indicate that PET has the potential to identify patients who will not response to therapy very early and might therefore be useful to optimize selection of treatment protocols [17,24,26].

Besides FDG-PET could be helpful to differentiate malignant from inflammatory lesions, in particular CNS-lymphoma from AIDS-related neurologic complications [27].
Prospective multicentric trials comparing PET with conventional techniques (CT, ultrasonography) are urgently needed to substantiate the cited preliminary data and to establish generally accepted indications for the use of PET. On the other hand, PET using radiolabelled amino or nucleinic acids appears to be an excellent technique for basic clinical research, e.g. evaluation of new cytostatic drugs. Biodistribution and metabolism of the latter might be examined after radiolabelling, too. Cooperation between nuclear medicine and oncology should therefore be stimulated.

Practical Considerations

In a clinical setting FDG is the radiopharmaceutical of choice to image malignant lymphoma. Due to the long physical half-life of ^{18}F, FDG is available in PET-centers as well as satellite-scanners being supplied from an external radiopharmacy. General use of FDG-PET in lymphoma patients seems therefore feasible. Depending on the clinical problem to be solved, PET should be performed as

- whole body procedure (staging or re-staging)

or

- static scan of selected body areas (evaluation of residual masses).

Whole body PET provides unique information about hypermetabolic foci throughout the body. Since measurement of attenuation coefficients is time-consuming if not performed during emission scanning, it might be dropped unless repeated studies for treatment control are planned. The latter should be quantitated by calculating differential uptake ratios (DUR) defined as [28]:

$$DUR = \frac{\text{tumor radioactivity / ml}}{\text{injected radioactivity / body weight}}$$

Dynamic scans including sequential collection of arterial or arterialized blood samples allow more sophisticated data analysis (Patlak-plot, parameter fitting) which is relevant for scientific studies. In clinical routine, however, impact of additional quantitative parameters still needs to be demonstrated. In contrast, advanced image processing, in particular iterative reconstruction may improve image quality and lesion detectability considerably. For accurate topographic interpretation of PET-scans image fusion with CT or MRI has proven to be useful and should be employed whenever possible. Table 3 summarizes the technical aspects of FDG-PET in lymphoma.

Table 3. FDG-PET in lymphoma - acquisition techniques.

Parameter	Static PET	Whole Body PET	Dynamic PET
patient preparation	12 hours fasting prior to FDG-injection		
radioactivity (MBq)	100-400[a]	100-400[a]	100-400[a]
attenuation correction	yes	optional	yes
scan begin[b]	45	30-45	immediate
scan duration[c]	10-15	5-15	variable
serum collection	-	-	mandatory
quantitation	DUR	--/DUR[d]	k_i/MR_{glu}

[a] depending on type of detector
[b] minutes following injection
[c] minutes per bed position
[d] in case of attenuation correction

abbreviations:
DUR - differential uptake ratio
k_i - influx constant for FDG
MR_{glu} - glucose metabolic rate (LC = 1)

Conclusion

Based on the clinical studies so far available FDG-PET appears to have great potential to improve staging and treatment control in malignant lymphoma. If these results can be substantiated in larger trials, PET might become part of the routine diagnostic workup in lymphoma and replace some of the imaging techniques currently used. Using other compounds (radiolabelled amino acids, nucleinic acids, chemotherapeutic drugs) PET is an extremely powerful tool for clinical research in oncology which should become better known among oncologists to be fully exploited.

References

1. Genereux GP, Howie JL. Normal mediastinal lymphnode size and number: CT and anatomic study. AJR 1984;142:1095-1100.
2. Müller NL, Webb WR, Gamsu G. Paratracheal lymphadenopathy: radiographic findings and correlation with CT. Radiology 1985;165:761-765.
3. McLaughlin A, Magee MA, Greenough R, et al.. Current role of gallium scanning in the management of lymphoma. Eur J Nucl Med 1990;16:755-771.
4. Iosilevsky G, Front D, Bettman L, Hardoff R, Ben-Arieh Y. Uptake of gallium-67 citrate and 2-H-3 deoxyglucose in the tumor model following chemotherapy and radiotherapy. J Nucl Med 1985;26:278-282.
5. Tumeh S, Rosenthal DS, Kaplan WD, English RJ, Holman BL. Lymphoma: evaluation with Ga-67 SPECT. Radiology 1987;164:111-114.
6. Front D, Bar-Shalom R, Epelbaum R, et al.. Early detection of lymphoma recurrence by gallium-67 scintigraphy. J Nucl Med 1993;34:2101-2104.
7. Kostakogu L, Yeh SDJ, Portlock C, et al.. Validation of gallium-67-citrate single-photon emission computed tomography in biopsy-confirmed residual Hodgkin's disease in the mediastinum. J Nucl Med 1992;33:345-350.
8. Johannsson L, Mattsson S, Nosslin B, Leide-Svegborn S. Effective dose from radiopharmaceuticals. Eur J Nucl Med 1992;19:933-938.
9. Bares R, Galonska P, Dempke W, Handt St., Büll U, Osieka R. Somatostatin receptor scintigraphy in malignant lymphoma: first results and comparison with glucose metabolism measured by positron emission tomography. Horm Metab Res 1993;27(suppl):56-58.
10. Lipp RW, Silly H, Ranner G, et al.. Radiolabeled octreotide for the demonstration of somatostatin receptors in malignant lymphoma and lymphadenopathy. J Nucl Med 1995;36:13-18.
11. Reubi JC, Waser B, van Hagen M, et al.. In vitro and in vivo detection of somatostatin receptors in human malignant lymphomas. Int J Cancer 1992;50:895-900.
12. Sehweil AM, McKillop JH, Milroy R, et al.. ^{201}Tl scintigraphy in the staging of lung cancer, breast cancer, and lymphoma. Nucl Med Commun 1990;11:263-269.
13. Piwnica-Worms D, Chiu ML, Budding M, Kronauge JF, Kramer RA, Croop JM. Functional imaging of multidrug-resistant P-glycoprotein with an organotechnetium complex. Cancer Res 1993;53:977-984.
14. Dimitrakopoulou-Strauss A, Strauss LG, Goldschmidt H, Lorenz WJ, van Kaick G. PET with FDG and SPECT with Tc-99m-sestamibi for therapy management in patients with treated malignant lymphomas. J Nucl Med 1994;35:231P.
15. Paul R. Comparison of fluorine-18-2-Fluorodeoxyglucose and gallium-67 citrate imaging for detection of lymphoma. J Nucl Med 1987;28:288-292.
16. Okada J, Yoshikawa K, Imazeki K, et al.. The use of FDG-PET in the detection and management of malignant lymphoma: correlation of uptake with prognosis. J Nucl Med 1991;32:686-691.
17. Okada J, Yoshikawa K, Itami M, et al.. Positron emission tomography using fluorine-18-fluorodeoxyglucose in malignant lymphoma: a comparison with proliferative activity. J Nucl Med 1992; 33: 325-329.
18. Leskinen-Kallio S, Ruotsalainen U, Nagren K, Teräs M, Joensuu H. Uptake of carbon- 11-methionine and fluorodeoxyglucose in non-Hodgkin's lymphoma: a PET study. J Nucl Med 1991;32:1211-1218.

19. Schönberger JA, Stollfuß JC, Kocher F, et al.. Whole body 18-FDG-PET for staging of malignant lymphomas. Eur J Nucl Med 1994;21:727.
20. Hoh CK, Glaspy JA, Hawkins RA, et al.. Utility of whole body PET in the staging of Hodgkin's disease and lymphoma. J Nucl Med 1994;35:221P.
21. Newman JS, Francis IR, Kaminski MS, Wahl RL. Imaging of lymphomawith PET with 2-(F-18)-Fluoro-2-deoxy-D-glucose: Correlation with CT. Radiology 1994;190: 111-116.
22. Bares R, Altehoefer C, Cremerius U, et al.. FDG-PET for metabolic classification of residual lymphoma masses after chemotherapy. J Nucl Med 1994;35:131P.
23. Garcia JR, Kim EE, Wong FCL, et al.. Ga-67 citrate scan in the differentiation of bone lymphoma from post-treatment changes: comparison with FDG-PET scan. J Nucl Med 1994;35:131P.
24. Hoekstra OS, Ossenkoppele GJ, Golding R, et al.. Early treatment response in malignant lymphoma, as determined by planar Fluorine-18-Fluorodeoxyglucose scintigraphy. J Nucl Med 1993;34:1706-1710.
25. Martiat Ph, Ferrant A, Labar D, et al.. In vivo measurement of carbon-11 thymidine uptake in non-Hodgkin's lymphoma using positron emission tomography. J Nucl Med 1988;29:1633-1637.
26. Kubota K, Ishiwata K, Kubota R, et al.. Tracer feasibility for monitoring tumor radiotherapy: a quadruple tracer study with fluorine-18-fluorodeoxyglucose, or fluorine-18-fluorodeoxyuridine, L[methyl-^{14}C]methionine, [6-^{3}H]thymidine, and gallium-67. J Nucl Med 1991;32:2118-2123.
27. Hoffman JM, Waskin HA, Schifter T, et al.. FDG-PET in differentiating lymphoma from nonmalignant central nervous system lesions in patients with AIDS. J Nucl Med 1993;34:567-575.
28. Woodard HQ, Gigler RE, Freed B, Russ G. Expression of tissue isotope distribution. J Nucl Med 1975;16:958-959.

8

WHOLE BODY POSITRON EMISSION TOMOGRAPHY IN ONCOLOGY

Ulrich Feine, Roland Lietzenmayer, Wolfgang Müller-Schauenburg

It has been shown in numerous studies that malignant tumors can be identified by increased trapping of ^{18}F fluorodeoxyglucose (FDG) [1]. The reported sensitivity of positron-emission-tomography (PET) with FDG varies between 80-90%. Until 1993 the maximum field of view (FOV) of commercially available PET-scanners was 5-10 cm confining the use of PET to defined body regions. Recently high resolution PET-scanners with 15 cm FOV have been developed. Sequential scanning of 5-11 FOV's allows to perform whole body (WB) scans - head to knee or head to foot - in 30-55 minutes (Fig.1) taking maximum profit of the favourable properties of FDG for tumor diagnosis and staging.

Whole Body PET in Tuebingen

In January 1994 a PET-scanner with 15.2 cm FOV (ADVANCE, General Electrics Medical Systems) was established in the Department of Nuclear Medicine/Eberhard-Karls-University Tübingen, and since that time systematically used for WB-PET studies in malignant tumors. PET-scans were performed parallel to computed tomography (CT), magnetic resonance imaging (MRI), and ultrasonography. Diagnostic results were retrospectively evaluated in cooperation with radiologists and clinicians involved in the studies.
A total of 425 PET-examinations has been performed during 1994, 375 as WB-PET in oncological patients. FDG was used in 357 examinations (injected dose: 5 MBq/kg body weight, 18 hrs. fasting prior to PET), in 16 studies ^{18}F fluoride (FF; injected dose: 5 MBq/kg body weight) was injected for imaging of bone metastases. Transmission scans for attenuation correction and quantitation of ^{18}F distribution were obtained in 92 studies. Due to limitations of scanning time, all other patients were investigated by emission scans only. The entire acquisition protocol is demonstrated in Table 1.

R. Bares and G. Lucignani (eds.) Clinical PET, 75–83.

Table 1. Acquisition protocol of FDG-PET (begin: 30-45 minutes after injection)

scan	field of view (cm)	duration (min.)
emission (1 FOV)	15	5-7
whole-body (head to knee)	75-100 (5-7 FOV)	25-35
whole-body (head to feet)	180 (12 FOV)	60-80
transmission (1 FOV)	5	5
whole-body (head to knee)	75	25

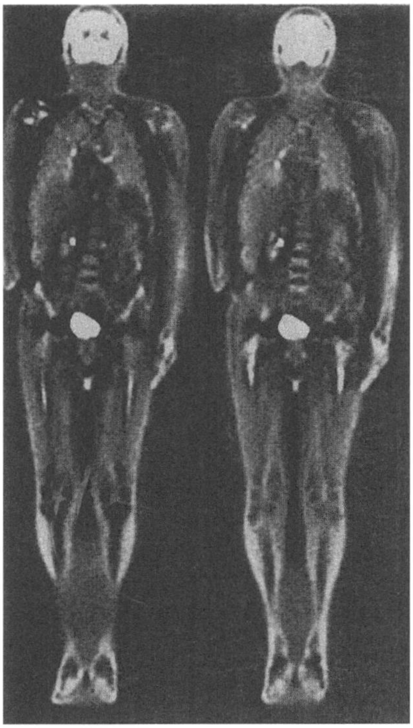

Figure 1. FDG WB-PET (no attenuation correction) in a 7 yrs. old male with multiple metastases (bone, lymphnodes) of an unknown primary tumor later identified as malignant non-Hodgkin lymphoma.

Time might be saved by measuring transmission after emission data. this feature has become possible by recently developed commercial software packages. Further improvements, however, are still desirable to reduce the scanning time and subsequently increase the patient throughput (e.g. simultaneous emission and transmission scanning, use of predefined attenuation coefficients). The patient groups studied so far are listed in Table 2.

Table 2. Patients investigated by FDG- or FF-PET

diagnosis	examinations	patients
malignant melanoma	84	70 (3 FF)
ocular melanoma	8	7
malignant lymphoma	56	49
breast cancer	45	44 (4 FF)
thyroid carcinoma	37	31
various malignancies (35 types)	119	103 (9 FF)

The large group of patients suffering from various types of malignant tumors was studied to get an overview about the clinical utility of FDG WB-PET in oncology. FF-PET was performed in 16 patients because of suspected bone metastases (melanoma, breast cancer, prostatic cancer, lung cancer) or primary osteosarcoma.

Diagnostic Results

MALIGNANT MELANOMA

FDG-PET was performed for detection of lymphnode or distant metastases and retrospectively compared with findings of CT and MRI-studies obtained within less than 3 weeks. The results were analyzed with regard to findings in identical FOV´s (PET vs CT/MRI) or additional findings of WB-PET. Furthermore a lesion-by-lesion analysis of PET and CT was made in 25 patients with more than 150 metastases to determine the critical size of lesions still visible in PET.

The complete work-up of all PET-findings revealed an overall sensitivity of 87%, specificity of 75%, accuracy of 85%, and positive predictive value of 87%. In comparison to CT (identical FOV), PET detected additional lesions in 19 patients, mainly lymphnode, liver, or bone metastases. WB PET-scans disclosed unknown metastases in 9 further patients. False negative PET-findings were obtained in 7 patients and are probably due to small size (diameter: <8 mm) although histological confirmation of most of these lesions could not be achieved. False positive findings were obtained in 4 patients: 4 (probably 7) inflammatory lymphnodes, 1 benign breast focus, and 6 bone or lung lesions not verified by CT or MRI.

Eight WB PET-studies with attenuaton correction of the facial skull were performed in 7 patients with known ocular melanoma before and after local ^{125}I or Ruthenium implants. All melanomas exceeding 8 mm in diameter were correctly visualized while a choreoideal melanoma of 2-8 mm was missed because of poor FDG-uptake. Additional WB-PET showed extraocular metastases (lung, liver, brain [previously unknown]) in one patient. Repeated scans revealed enhanced FDG-uptake 3 weeks after irradiation (flare effect?) while in another patient 6 months after irradiation no significant FDG-accumulation could be demonstrated. Systematic follow-up studies are ongoing.

MALIGNANT LYMPHOMA

WB-PET was performed as a part of staging or re-staging procedures in patients with Hodgkin´s disease (n=17), non-Hodgkin lymphomas (n=17), MALT (Mucosa

Associated Lymphatic Tissue) lymphomas (n=1), TALL (T-cell Acute Lymphatic Leukemia) lymphomas (n=1), and 4 patients with not classified malignant lymphomas. Direct comparison of PET-findings with CT revealed a sensitivity of 92%, specificity of 75%, accuracy of 88%, and a positive predictive value of 94%. PET was able to demonstrate 9 unknown lymphoma manifestations (cervical nodes: n=4, hilar nodes: n=3, bone lesions: n=1, soft tissue lesions: n=1). FDG-uptake in untreated patients was extremely high allowing for excellent tumor/non-tumor contrast. Follow up PET-studies (n=6) showed normal FDG-distribution in patients with complete remission (Fig.1) while otherwise hypermetabolic nodules remained visible.
Negative PET-findings were obtained in 3 patients presenting residual masses after chemotherapy. Since no histological confirmation is available, it is still unclear whether they are false or true negative (absence of viable lymphoma). False positive results were due to inflammatory lymphnodes (n=1) or adenomas of the thyroid (n=2).

BREAST CANCER AND OTHER GYNECOLOGICAL TUMORS

Twenty patients with suspected breast cancer were investigated preoperatively. The results of PET are summarized in Table 3. False negative findings were obtained in 3 small tumors (ductal carcinoma: diameter 10/22 mm, lobular carcinoma: diameter 12 mm) which did not show enhanced FDG-accumulation compared to surrounding breast tissue. The only false negative lymphnode metastasis was also less than 10 mm in diameter. Fig.2 shows the WB-PET of a primary breast carcinoma with axillary lymphnode metastases.

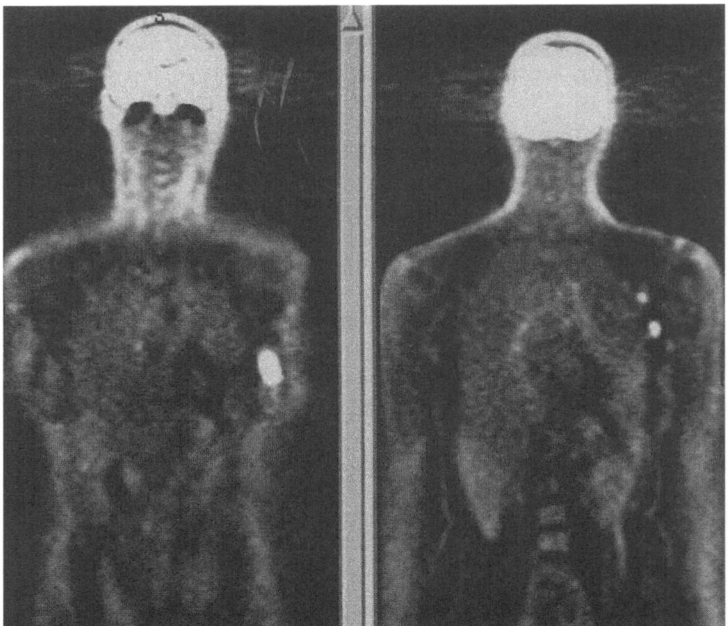

Figure 2. FDG WB-PET in a 45-yrs old female with suspected breast cancer. PET reveals high FDG-uptake in the primary tumor as well as lymphnode metastases (confirmed by surgery)

Table 3. Results of FDG-PET in primary breast cancer

Lesion	n	sensitivity (%)	specificity (%)	accuracy (%)	PPV (%)
Primary tumors	20	75	90	81	90
Limphnode metastases	35	94	100	95	100

PPV = Positive predictive value

PET-scans in 20 patients with treated breast cancer revealed identical findings compared to CT except for 2 patients with lung metastases smaller than 8 mm shown by helical CT. In 8 patients with different gynecological tumors (chorioncarcinoma, 4 carcinomas of the cervix uteri, 2 ovarian carcinomas, 1 vaginal cancer) lymphnode as well as lung or adrenal metastases were correctly visualized by PET. One recurrent ovarian cancer was missed probably due to the small lesion size (microscopic infiltrations at the borderline of a scar area).

THYROID CARCINOMA

Thirty-seven PET-studies in 31 patients with differentiated thyroid cancer (papillary: n=8, follicular: n=17 including 2 oncocytic carcinomas, medullary: n=4) all having been treated by thyroidectomy and ^{131}I elimination of residual thyroid tissue have been performed because of suspected tumor recurrence (increased thyroglobuline or calcitonine levels). Results of the complete diagnostic work-up including ^{131}I scintigraphy (except for medullary thyroid carcinoma), bone and ^{201}Tl scintigraphy, CT, MRI, and ultrasonography were available in all patients and compared with the findings of WB-PET. After analyzing the metabolic behaviour (FDG vs ^{131}I) of metastases systematically we discovered a particular phenomenon we would like to call "Flipflop" (flipflop = electronic device or circuit capable of taking one of two stable states): metastases trapping ^{131}I showed no or only poor FDG-uptake while ^{131}I accumulation in metastases trapping FDG was weak or even missing. Thus, 4 different types of metabolic behaviour (FDG/^{131}I) could be separated:

type 1: FDG-positive / ^{131}I-negative;
type 2: FDG-negative / ^{131}I-positive
type 3: FDG-positive / ^{131}I-negative or
FDG negative / ^{131}I-positive (Fig.3)
type 4: FDG- and ^{131}I-positive (mainly low uptake)

Type 4 is probably caused by tumors composed of both well and less differentiated cells. In patients who were negative in PET and ^{131}I scintigraphy the combined use of all usual diagnostic procedures did not yield any evidence of a tumor recurrence. Table 4 correlates metabolic behaviour and histological type of thyroid cancer.

Table 4. Comparison of metabolism and histology of thyroid cancer

histology	type 1	type 2	type 3	type 4	all
papillary	5	1	2	2	10
follicular	8	4	2	1	15
oncocytic	3	0	0	1	4
total	16	5	4	4	29

In all patients with increased serum thyroglobuline without pathological findings of ^{131}I scintigraphy, FDG-PET was positive (sensitivity: 100 %), among them 6 patients with inconclusive outcome after routinee diagnostic work-up. Increased FDG-uptake was also found in 5 patients with follicular adenomas while no toxic adenoma was positive in PET.

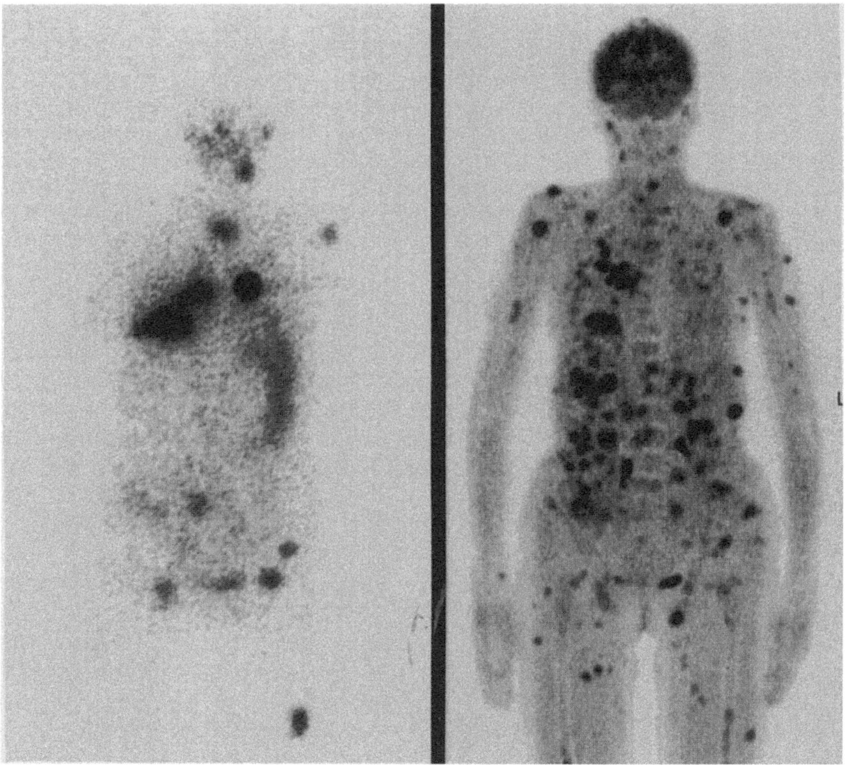

Fig. 3. Radioiodide WB-scans (left) and FDG WB-PET (sinogram projection; right) in a 63-yrs old female patient with papillary thyroid cancer and multiple lung and bone metastases revealing either I-131 or FDG uptake

VARIOUS MALIGNANCIES

In addition to the above mentioned 4 main tumor groups 119 WB PET-scans were performed in 103 patients suffering from a variety of malignant tumors (lung cancer, GEP-tumors, hepatocellular carcinoma, renal carcinoma, neuroblastoma, pancreatic cancer, prostatic cancer, sarcomas, colorectal cancer, thymomas, metastatic cancer of unknown origin). We found elevated FDG uptake in the majority of lesions allowing for correct PET diagnosis. False negative findings were obtained in 4 out of 8 hepatocellular carcinomas, a patient with Kaposi sarcoma and diffuse bone marrow-, liver-, and spleen infiltration, and 1 out of 9 neuroblastomas all positive in MIBG-scintigraphy (highly differentiated tumor?). There were only a few false positive results due to inflammatory disease or benign thyroid nodules.

WHOLE BODY FLUORIDE PET

Compared to the bone scintigraphy the sensitivity of FF-WB-PET for detecting bone metastases was markedly higher. The same was true when comparing FDG- and FF-PET (Fig. 4). Besides superior image quality and tumor contrast FF-PET allows for quantitative evaluation of bone metabolism which might gain clinical relevance used for treatment control (bone tumors), evaluation of surgical procedures (viability of bone transplants), or osteoporosis.

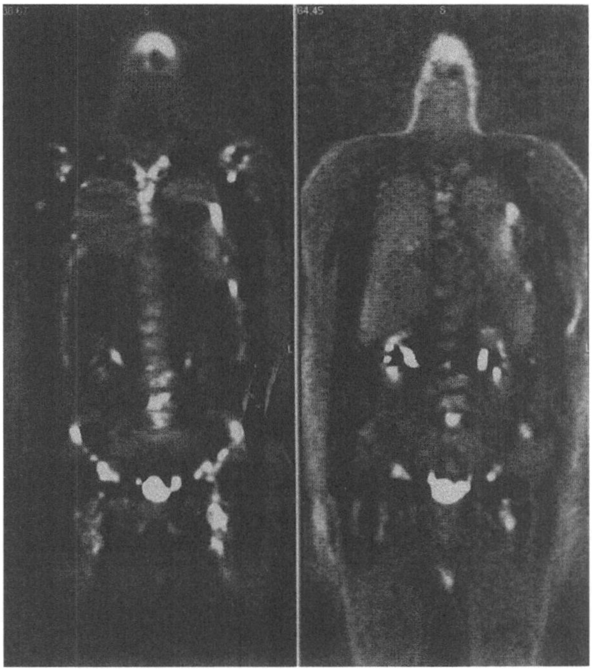

Fig. 4. FDG (left) and FF (right) WB-PET in a 63 year old male patient with multiple metastases of an unknown primary tumor.

Discussion

The first reports about WB-PET in oncology emerged in 1992 [2,3]. Since that time an increasing number of papers has been published stressing the high diagnostic sensitivity and clinical relevance of this new imaging technique [4-6]. Our experience confirms these results in a total of 304 patients with malignant tumors. The overall sensitivity of PET was in the range of 80-90 %, the specificity, accuracy, and positive predictive value was about 90 %. False negative findings were confined to tumors less than 8 mm in diameter, mainly lung metastases. False positive results were obtained in inflammatory lymphnodes, abscesses, and benign thyroid nodules. Furthermore FDG-uptake appeared

to be correlated to tumor differentiation in terms that high uptake is present in undifferentiated tumors and vice versa.
Analyzing the different tumor types in detail we found excellent results in malignant melanoma as recently reported by Yao and coworkers [7]. Compared to other imaging modalities PET allows for whole-body surveys within one study and may therefore be cost-effective when used as initial staging test. In case of ocular melanoma PET offers the opportunity for non-invasive tumor classification (benign vs malignant) as well as for staging or treatment control. However, large prospective studies are still needed to substantiate this initial clinical evaluation. Malignant lymphomas are characterized by very intense FDG-accumulation, too, and therefore easily detected by PET. Thus, WB-PET might be used as initial procedure for staging or re-staging, perhaps followed by CT or MR for morphological classification of metabolic abnormalities.
In breast cancer WB-PET allowed for accurate preoperative diagnosis of regional lymphnode metastases (sensitivity: 94%) while results in suspected primary tumors were less satisfactory (sensitivity: 75%). The clinical impact of FDG-PET for the diagnosis of breast cancer is therefore still uncertain. It may gain importance in advanced stages (T_3/T_4) to exclude distant metastases, if diagnostic accuracy of PET is shown to be significantly higher compared to routine imaging techniques.
Until now only few reports have been published dealing with FDG-PET in benign or malignant thyroid disease [8-11]. Our findings about alternative uptake of FDG or ^{131}I have not been published so far and may give new insights in the biology of differentiated thyroid cancer. Based upon our data it can be assumed that high uptake of ^{131}I in the presence of missing FDG-accumulation is indicative for a good prognosis while the inverse pattern may be associated with progressive disease. No interaction between FDG-uptake and the TSH-level has been noted so far. A similar correlation between glucose metabolism and differentiation has been described in brain tumors [12] and was noticed by us in neuroblastomas, too (highly differentiated ganglioneuromas are FDG-negative, but MIBG-positive).

Conclusion

Based upon our experience the major advantage of WB-PET with FDG compared to other imaging techniques is the combination of high tumor contrast (characteristic although not specific for cancer), a large FOV (whole body surveys possible), and relatively short examination periods (60-120 min., without transmission scanning: 35-60 min.). In future PET might be used for evaluation of tumor spread and treatment control, in particular in case of malignant lymphoma, lung cancer, or malignant melanoma. If PET will become the initial imaging procedure, the use of CT or MRI could be confined to patients with pathological PET results.
Diagnostic algorithms like the one mentioned might reduce the costs for diagnosis as was proposed recently [7]. One has to be aware, however, that the spatial resolution of modern PET-Scanners (8-10 mm) is still inferior to helical-CT although the clinical relevance of lesions smaller than 8mm has not been defined so far.
Attenuation correction is a prerequisite for quantitative PET. For screening of cancer it appears to be less important as was shown by comparing 74 attenuation-corrected PET-scans with the original, non-corrected tomograms. Thus, we believe that attenuation correction is desirable by principle, diagnostic accuracy, however, is not hampered by leaving it to selected clinical problems (e.g. the head and neck area).

References

1. Strauss LG, Conti PS. The application ofPET in clinical oncology.J.Nucl.Med. 1991, 32: 623-648.
2. Tse NY, Hawkins RA, Zimmer MJ, Dahlbaum M, et al 1992.:The application of positron emission tomography imaging with fluorodeoxygluose to the evaluation of breast disease. AnnSurg 1992, 216(1): 27-34.
3. Hawkins RA, Hoh C, Glapsy J, et al and Phelps ME: The role of positron emissiontomography in oncology and other whole body application. Sem.Nucl.Med. 22(4)1992: 268-284.
4. Hoh CK, Hawkins RA, Glaspy JA, Dahlborn M, Tse NY, et al: Cancer detection withwhole body PET using 18 F-fluoro-deoxyclucose. J.Comp.Assist.Tomogr. 1993; 17(4): 582-589.
5. Rege SD, Hoh CK, Glapsy JA, Aberle DR, Dahlbom M et al.: Imaging of pulmonarymass lesions with whole body positron emission tomography and fluorodeoxyglucose.Cancer 1993: 1, 72(1) 82-90.
6. Karlan BY, Hawkins R, Hoh CK, Lee M et al: Whole body positron emission tomography with 2-18 F fluor-desoxyglucose can detect recurrent ovarian carcinoma. Gynecol. Oncol 1993, 51 (2): 175-181.
7. Yao WJ, Hoh CK, Glapsy JA, et al: Whole body FDG PET imaging for staging ofmalignant melanoma. J.NuclMed. 1994; 34: 8P.
8. Joensuu H, Ahonen A.Imaging ofmetastases ofthyroid carcinoma with fluorine-18-fluoro-deoxyglucose. J.Nucl.Med. 1987, 28: 910-914.
9. Joensuu H, Ahonen A, Klemi PJ.18-F-fluorodeoxyglucose imaging in preoperativediagnosis of thyroid malignancy. Eur.J.Nucl.Med. 1988, 13: 502-506.
10. Schmidt D, Herzog H, Langen KJ, Müller-Gärtner HW. Glucose metabolism in thyroid cancer metastases. A pilot study using 18-fluoro-2-deoxyglucose and positron emission tomography. Exp.Clin.Endocrinol. 1994, 102: 51-54.
11. Börner AR, Voth E, Schicha H. 18-FDG-PET bei Patienten mit immunogener Hyper thyreose vor Radiojodtherapie. Nucl.Med. 1994, 33 A 81.
12. Di Chiro G. Positron emission tomography using 18-F-fluorodeoxyglucose in brain tumors. A powerful diagnostic and prognostic tool. Invest.Radiol. 1987, 22: 360-371.

Part Three:
PET in Neurology

9

PET IN NEUROLOGY - CLINICAL PROBLEMS

Cornelius Weiller

Positron emission tomography (PET) is continouing to have a major scientific impact on clinical neurology. Its role in routine clinical practice has been restricted by the lack of prospective studies on a large number of patients, mainly due to the restricted availability of PET centres at clinical institutions with access to appropriate patient data bases. However, recent progress has been made in several areas, which should stimulate the formulation of new questions, in which PET might be of major value.

Cerebrovascular Diseases

Potential applications of PET in stroke are listed in Table 1. PET has considerably improved our knowledge of the pathophysiology of stroke and the mechanisms by which the brain reacts to decreased perfusion pressure [1]. The study of acute stroke is still the most interesting and promising aspects. Every year 160.000 germans suffer from stroke, and about half of them will be unable to return to work again. Thus, stroke has a major socio-economic impact. Pathophysiology of acute stroke is changing, because with the application of thrombolytic therapy in acute stroke, many more cases with early reperfusion are encountered. In the decisive time frame, the first 6-12 hours after the insult, no conclusive PET data on large numbers of patients are available. However, today PET is the only instrument which is able to give the necessary information on rCBF, $rCMRO_2$, OEF, rCBV, necessary for therapeutic decisions [2]. The effects of ischemia on the brain depend on the severity of ischemia, the duration of ischemia, determined by the time until recanalisation of the occluded vessel occurs and by the vulnerability of the tissue, high for neurons, low for glial cells.
Aggressive therapeutic approaches in stroke are based on the assumption of potentially reversible damaged tissue, the so called penumbra. It is still unclear whether a penumbra really exists in man. Theoretically, a penumbral state can develop into three different conditions. Rapid re-establishment of sufficient perfusion results in restitutio ad integrum (a probable mechanism underlying TIAs). In permanent occlusion or very low blood flow values, penumbra will rapidly progress into frank infarction. From animal studies and some experience in human stroke, a third way seems to exist, which is becoming increasingly common with the early reperfused cases of today, i.e. incomplete infarction or selective neuronal loss [3-5]. This does occur in areas with critically lowered rCBF, which is just enough for the robust glial cells, thereby sparing the macroscopic shape, however not sufficient for the neurons with their high metabolic

R. Bares and G. Lucignani (eds.) Clinical PET, 87–91.

demand, causing loss of function. The extent and severity of incomplete infarction largely affects the prognosis and rehabilitation, as restoration of function is dependent on the spared parts of the network underlying the observed function.

Probably the best current example in human strokes are striatocapsular infarcts. These are purely subcortical infarcts with intact shape of the overlying cortex on structural imaging. They are due to occlusion of the middle cerebral artery (MCA) at the M1-segment, with the cortex being irrigated by leptomeningeal collaterals [6]. Approximately half of these patients present with neurological dysfunction that must be attributed to the cortex, e.g.; aphasia, which is due to incomplete (and as such not visible on initial CT scanning) infarction. These cortical symptoms correlate with a longer duration of MCA occlusion and poor collateral blood flow [4]. In these cases, cortical rCBF does not normalise as would be expected in functional deactivation ("Diaschisis") but the hypoperfusion deepens and correlates with a focal atrophy on MRI, suggesting selective neuronal loss of the cerebral cortex during the acute phase. There are several scientific aspects of potential PET studies: a) how deep and for how long must ischemia be present before a complete or incomplete infarction appears? b) What are the functional and structural consequences of early and late reperfusion ? And c) how can symptoms without any morphological correlate in the acute phase be differentiated from true "functional disconnections". But there are also direct clinical implications, as the extent of incomplete infarction has direct implications for the prognosis of the patient. The process of recovery is influenced by the number of surviving neurons. With growing financial pressures on rehabilitation services, difficult decisions may have to be taken as to which patients should receive such therapy. A recent study showed how incomplete infarction can easily be differentiated from functional deactivation by comparing rCBF measurements (^{15}O) and [^{11}C]Flumazenil scans in a MCA occlusion model in baboons [7]. Flumazenil, as a marker of the central benzodiazepine receptor site as part of the ubiquitous GABA receptor complex, can be used as a tracer to estimate neuronal density [8]. All baboons had striatocapsular infarcts. While in some cortical areas Flumazenil-uptake was unchanged in hypoperfused cortical areas, suggesting functional deactivation without neuronal loss, in others hypoperfusion was paralleled by a decrease in Flumazenil-uptake, indicating loss of neurons in a macroscopically intact cerebral cortex.

Several PET activation studies in the last two years have demonstrated that brain function is highly adaptable after stroke [9-12]. A complex pattern of reorganisation in the motor as well as the language system has been found in patients who recovered from a stroke despite persisting destruction of responsible fields and tracts. Further studies will have to be done to elucidate the precise mechanisms underlying this reorganisation and enable its implementation in rehabilitation concepts. The future of activation studies clearly lies in the integration of the different methods to combine the high spatial resolution of anatomical MRI and the sensitivity of PET with the high time resolution of MEG or MRI-spectroscopy [13]. Functional magnetic resonance imaging, though promising, however, is still in its infancy and at the moment, it is unclear whether it will ever be able to replace PET in activation studies.

Progressive stroke and the discussion whether or not increased blood pressure after stroke should be treated promises to become another thrilling topic. About 30-40% of all strokes progress, having a major impact on the duration of hospital stay, and discharge to nursing institutions instead of home and resulting in markedly increased costs [14]. Autoregulation, which keeps rCBF constant over a wide range of blood pressure variations under normal conditions, is impaired in stroke [15]. The infarcted brain is unable to regulate its own blood supply in the acute phase and cerebral perfusion follows the systemic blood pressure passively. In a recent study 113 out of 868 stroke

patients had a progressive stroke with development of new symptoms within the first 36 hours. Out of 22 parameters studied, systolic blood pressure on admission (inverse relation) and diabetes were the only discriminatory factors [14]. PET can be a most valuable tool to assess the mechanisms behind the assumption that increased blood pressure should not be lowered after stroke.
In secondary stroke prevention PET does not seem to have a role. Prognosis following a second stroke is not related to rCBF/rCBV or rOEF [16]. Only a small percentage of strokes is due to hemodynamic failure [17]. The two large trials on carotid endarterectomy have clearly demonstrated that symptomatic stenoses, greater 70%, should be operated on, regardless of intracranial hemodynamics [18]. Unsettled is the question, whether a carotid artery stenosis should be operated when the contralateral side is occluded but still produces further symptoms. Assessment of hemodynamics that does not require side to side comparisons clearly could help here. New techniques for the assessment of hemodynamic alteration using MRI are emerging [19, 20].

Dementia

Dementia imposes an increasing socio-economic hardship on our society. According to a US survey, 4% of the over 65 year olds and 30 % of the over 85 year olds suffer from dementia causing an annual cost of $ 44 billion/year for care. Alzheimer's disease accounts for almost 50% of all dementia cases. Clinical diagnosis is easy in advanced cases, however, is often ambigous in the early course of the disease. Assessment of glucose metabolism with [^{18}F]FDG-PET is the ideal tool to identify characteristic patterns of hypometabolism in early cases [21]. All autoptic verifications of the 500 Alzheimer patients studied by PET so far, proved to be correct. One PET procedure can help avoid the repetition of many costly procedures as MRI. The family or individuals at risk in familial Alzheimer can be advised and PET may represent an ideal criterium to control therapeutic effects. There is a subform of dementia, which is difficult to diagnose, in which intellectual decline is preceded by isolated and progressive neuropsychological deficits. Here [^{18}F]FDG-PET, again is the ideal tool to show discrete patterns of hypometabolism as an explanation for the observed clinical findings. Vascular dementia is very frequent as well and accounts for 30-40% of all dementia cases. It consists mainly of Binswangers disease, characterised by multiple small lacunas and periventricular demyelination. Diagnosis is made clinically and with CT or MRI. There is no role for PET here [22]. The term "multi infarct dementia" should not be used anymore, as it implies an incorrect pathophysiological background and has been excluded from the new classification [23].

Epilepsy

The role of PET in the routine assessment of epileptics is widely discussed. Epilepsy is a very common disease. About 800.000 patients in Germany have active epilepsy, 20% of which have fits resistant to drug treatment and should be further evaluated, possibly for surgery, as this can lead to significant improvement in about 60 % of highly selected cases. However, this number is much too high for the few epilepsy centres to cope with. Several methods are offered to find the epileptic foci for presurgical evaluation. All of these have to be tested against the only valid gold standard, which is considerable improvement without any persisting deficits after surgery. When weighing the different methods, it has to be kept in mind that epileptic seizures, although often starting at one site in the brain, most often generalise within milliseconds. Obviously, methods with a time resolution of seconds or even minutes are unable to mirror the events during fits adequately. Semiology, i.e. the clinical description of symptoms together with high resolution MRI (different sequences in planes perpendicular to the temporal lobe, T2-SE, inversion recovery) gives good clues in most cases, besides being non-invasive. Best results can be obtained by recording ictal-EEG's using implanted depth-electrodes. However this is a costly, invasive and time-consuming procedure. Moreover, location of the implantation must be guided by external clues. If there is disagreement, [^{18}F]FDG-PET is often able to show hypometabolic areas, which are not detected by MRI, especially in the medial temporal cortex [24, 25]. It seems too early to renounce to ictal-EEG recordings in cases, in which MRI and PET are conformative [24, 26]. Further clues can be gained from a state of the art neuropsychological examination. As there are no definitve controlled studies, this is a very personal view, that is not shared by others. As different neurotransmitters are involved in epileptic seizures, ligand studies are principally able to localise the pathophysiological changes. There is one study using [^{11}C]-Flumazenil as a ligand for the central benzodiazepine receptor site that showed a focus of decreased flumazenil binding within hypometabolic regions, as defined by [^{18}F]FDG-PET [27]. An important role for PET in neurosurgery may be its support for the neurosurgeon by identifying areas to be spared by an operation (e.g.; language or motor centres) [28]. PET activation and fMRI studies should be compared with the gold standard of today, the Wada-test , which has the complication rate of cerebral angiographies. First results suggest some disagreement with the functional imaging techniques having more sensitivity.

While PET has a wide potential in the research of the diseases of the human brain, much work still has to be done before PET can be seen as a routine tool, supported by the national health authorities. What could be the future prospects of clinical PET in neurology ? 1)Prospective studies using statistical valid methods and a large group of patients and adequate controls dedicated to address defined clinical questions, 2) a flow independent tracer of neuronal density, 3) in the long run, the labelling of therapeutic drugs. All this can be successful only in a concerted action between nuclear medicine physicians, radiochemists, cyclotron / PET operators and physicians running daily clinics.

References

1. Powers WJ. Cerebral hemodynamics in ischemic cerebrovascular disease. Ann Neurol 1991; 29:231-240.
2. Heiss WD, Herholz K. Assessment of pathophysiology of stroke by positron emission tomography. European Journal of Nuclear Medicine 1994; 21:455-465.
3. Lassen NA, Olsen TS, Hqjgaard K, Skriver E. Incomplete infarction: A CT negative irreversible ischemic brain lesion. J Cereb Blood Flow Metab 1983; 3, suppl.1:S602-S603.
4. Weiller C, Willmes K, Reiche W, et al. The case of aphasia or neglect after striatocapsular infarction. Brain 1993; 116:1509-1525.
5. Garcia JH, Wagner S, Liu KF, Hu XJ. The neurologic deficit and the extent of neuronal necrosis attributable to middle cerebral artery occlusion. Stroke 1995; 26:(in press)
6. Weiller C, Ringelstein EB, Reiche W, Thron A, Buell U. The large striatocapsular infarct. A clinical and pathophysiological entity. Arch Neurol 1990; 47:1085-1091.

7. Sette G, Baron JC, Young AR, et al. In vivo mapping of brain benzodiazepine receptor changes by positron emission tomography after focal ischemia in the anesthetized baboon. Stroke 1993; 24:2046-2058.
8. Lassen NA, Bartenstein PA, Lammertsma AA, et al. Benzodiazepine Receptor Quantification In Vivo in Humans Using [11C]Flumazenil and PET: Application of the Steady-State Principle. J Cereb Blood Flow Metab 1995; 15:152-165.
9. Weiller C, Chollet F, Friston KJ, Wise RJS, Frackowiak RSJ. Functional reorganization of the brain in recovery from striatocapsular infarction in man. Ann Neurol 1992; 31:463-472.
10. Weiller C, Ramsay SC, Wise RJS, Friston KJ, Frackowiak RSJ. Individual patterns of functional reorganization in the human cerebral cortex after capsular infarction. Ann Neurol 1993; 33:181-189.
11. Rijntjes M, Weiller C, Krams M, Bauermann T, Diener HC, Faiss J. Functional Magnetic Resonance Imaging in Recovery from Motor Stroke. Stroke 1994; 25:256.(abstract)
12. Weiller C, Isensee Ch, Rijntjes M, et al. Recovery from Wernicke's aphasia - A PET study. Ann Neurol 1995; (in press)
13. Eulitz C, Elbert T, Bartenstein PA, Weiller C, Müller SP, Pantev C. Comparison of magnetic and metabolic brain activity during a verb generation task. NeuroReport 1994; 6:97-100.
14. Jørgensen HS, Nakayama H, Raaschou HO, Olsen TS. Effect of blood pressure and diabetes on stroke in progression. Lancet 1994; 344:156-159.
15. Powers WJ. Acute hypertension after stroke: The scientific basis for treatment decisions. Neurology 1993; 43:461-467.
16. Powers WJ, Tempel LW, Grubb RL. Influence of cerebral hemodynamics on stroke risk: one year follow-up of 30 medically treated patients. Ann Neurol 1989;25:325-30.
17. Weiller C, Ringelstein EB, Reiche W, Buell U. Clinical and hemodynamic aspects of low flow infarcts. Stroke 1991; 22:1117-1123.
18. Ad Hoc Committee American Heart Association. Guidelines for Carotid Endarterectomy. Stroke 1995; 26:188-201.
19. Vanninen R, Kolvisto K, Tulla H, Manninen J, Partanen K. Hemodynamic Effects of Carotid Endarterctomy by Magnetic Reson a nce Flow Quantification. Stroke 1995; 26:84-89.
20. Kleinschmidt A, Steinmetz H, Sitzer M, Merboldt K-D, Frahm J. Magnetic Resonance Imaging of Regional Cerebral Blood oxygenation changes under acetazolamine in carotid occlusive disease. Stroke 1995; 26:106-110.
21. Grady CL, Haxby JV, Horwitz B, et al. A longitudinal study of the early neuropsychological and cerebral metabolic changes in dementia of the Alzheimer type. J Clin Exp Neuropsychology 1987; 10:579-596.
22. Sabri O, Hellwig D, Kaiser HJ, et al. Einfluss morphologischer Veränderungen auf Durchblutung und Stoffwechsel bei zerebraler Mikroangiopathie. Nucl Med 1995;
23. McKhann G, Drachman D, Folstein M, Katzman R, Price D, Stadlan EM. Clinical diagnosis of Alzheimer's disease: report of the NINCDS- ADRDA work group under the auspices of Department of Health and Human Services Task Force on Alzheimer's disease. Neurology 1984; 34:939-944.
24. Spencer SS. The relative contributions of MRI, SPECT and PET Imaging in Epilepsy. Epilepsia 1994; 35 (suppl. 6):S72-S89.
25. Pawlik G, Fink GR, Kessler J, Heiss WD. PET and functional testing in temporal lobe epilepsy. Acta Neurol Scand 1994; Supplement 152:150-156.
26. Duncan JS. Discussion. Acta Neurol Scand 1994; Supplement 152:135-136.
27. Savic I, Persson A, Roland P, Pauli S, Sedvali G, Widen L. In vivo demonstration of reduced benzodiazepine receptor binding in human epileptic foci. Lancet 1988; 863.
28. Leblanc R, Meyer E, Bub D, Zatorre RJ, Evans AC. Language localization with activation positron emission tomography. Neurosurgery 1992; 31:369-373.

10

ASSESSMENT OF BRAIN TUMORS, CEREBROVASCULAR AND CEREBRAL DEGENERATIVE DISEASES WITH PET

Karl Herholz

The first clinical applications of positron emission tomography (PET) more than fifteen years ago were in neurology, mainly using the 2-[^{18}F]fluoro-2-deoxy-D-glucose ([^{18}F]FDG) technique derived from experimental autoradiographic work. Today, [^{18}F]FDG is still the preferred tracer for most clinical neurological studies because of the close relation between local cerebral glucose metabolism (lCMRGlu) and the density of functionally active synapses, which is most informative in a large variety of generalized and local functional brain disorders. Technical advantages include: high resolution images (due to low positron energy of Fluorine-18), low noise levels at low doses (with typical data acquisition time of 20-40 min at 185-370 MBq injected dose), little patient cooperation required, absolute quantitation without arterial puncture, tracer batch production possible (due to relatively long half-life time).

State-of-the-art tomographs should scan the whole brain without bed movement, provide similar high resolution (FWHM 6mm or less) in all three axes for 3D image reorientation, and perform accurate corrections for random counts, scatter, and attentuation to yield quantitative data for calculation of lCMRGlu. This provides a solid basis to determine regional normal values and confidence limits which are indispensable for objective data assessment, and represents the most essential difference from less reliable techniques, such as single photon emission tomography (SPET). Quantitative regional data analysis must supplement visual scan reading, which currently is the most efficient way to detect possible abnormalities, but whose validity in terms of sensitivity and specificity is severely limited by considerable subjective and arbitrary technical influences (e.g. selection of colour scales and background subtraction).

Three-dimensional coregistration with morphological tomographic data, X-ray computed tomography (CT) and magnetic resonance imaging (MRI) is possible now, although not yet widespread in clinical practice. Current experience suggests that it is a major step forward, comparable to the introduction of PET itself, that will substantially improve clinical and scientific data interpretation. It provides accurate information on the topography of abnormalities (which is essential for surgeons), permits much more detailed studies on the relation between variation of brain anatomy or brain lesions and their functional effects, and facilitates differentiation between reductions of regional brain activity due to atrophy (signal loss due to limited resolution and partial volume effects) versus actual reductions of functional tissue activity (per unit volume of tissue).

PET is rarely needed to establish a clinical neurological diagnosis. The same is true for other functional methods, e.g. electroencephalography and evoked potentials, but these are less expensive and therefore used more liberally. Yet, PET is currently the most

R. Bares and G. Lucignani (eds.) Clinical PET, 93–102.

versatile and accurate tool to investigate local changes of brain biochemistry, including transmitters and receptors, and functional activity that occur in neurological diseases, and therefore PET studies comprise a considerable part of the current international neurological literature. In the following chapters, I am going to demonstrate how PET often gives a more detailed and objective assessment of a patient's condition than traditional diagnostic techniques. Thus, it contributes significantly to a better understanding of the pathophysiology, functional consequences and course of brain diseases, and thus helps to devise new therapeutic strategies (which is particularly difficult in neurology).

Brain Tumors

Brain tumors account for approximately 1,5% of all new cancers, and for 2,2% of all cancer deaths [1]. Annual mortality is approximately 5 per 100 000 persons. In people under 35 years of age age they account for 8 to 22% of all cancer deaths. CT and MRI are standard imaging techniques for diagnosis of brain tumors and may also contribute to differentiation between tumor types. In special clinical situations, PET can answer specific questions (Tab. 1) and may thus improve treatment planning [2].

Table 1. Clinical issues and usefulness of PET in brain tumors

Clinical question	PET tracer	
	[^{18}F]FDG	amino acids
Diff. diagnosis: tumor vs. non-tumor	(+)[a]	(+)[b]
Diff. diagnosis: tumor type	-	-
Histological grade of malignancy	(+)[c]	(+)[d]
Prognosis of survival time	+	-
Tumor extent of low grade tumors	-	+
Localize areas of high cell density	+	?
Monitoring of therapy	(+)[e]	+
Distinction between recurrent tumor and radiation necrosis	(+)[e]	?

+: useful.
-: not useful.
?: insufficient available data.
(+) useful with significant limitations as explained below(a-d).
a) lesions with high [^{18}F]FDG uptake include: fresh abscesses, approx. 10% of recent ischemic infarcts, active epileptic foci; low [^{18}F]FDG uptake does not exclude tumor.
b) lesions with increased amino acid uptake include: recent reperfused ischemic infarcts, active inflammatory lesions; low amino acid uptake is rare in tumors.
c) correlations exist, but are weaker than for contrast enhancement with CT and MRI in gliomas.
d) differentiation between viable tumor and necrotic tissue is uncertain in areas with [^{18}F]FDG uptake less than in normal gray matter.

In human gliomas, which account for approximately 35% of all human brain tumors, tumor glucose consumption relative to contralateral brain CMRGlu is an indicator of clinical prognosis in terms of survival time [3-6]. This is apparently due to a tendency towards higher glucose consumption in tumors with higher histological malignancy [3] in combination with reduction of global cerebral CMRGlu in more aggressive and invasive tumors. Estimation of prognosis is of particular interest in patients with a histological diagnosis of low-grade astrocytoma, because survival times vary widely (few months to more than 10 years), bioptic tissue samples may not have been representative of the whole tumor, and there is considerable uncertainty about the best therapeutic management (waiting until clinical manifestation of tumor progression vs. early intervention) [7]. In this tumor type, glucose consumption correlates with cell density [8], and therefore "hot" tumor areas have been identified as good targets for stereotactic biopsy to improve its diagnostic yield [9].

Highly malignant cerebellar medulloblastomas often have very high glucose consumption rates [10]. There are reports that aggressiveness and growth rate of meningiomas is also related to glucose consumption [11,12]. Yet, benign pituitary adenomas may also show increased glucose consumption [13]. Clinical interpretation is uncertain in some rare glioma types: juvenile pilocytic astrocytomas (WHO grade 1) may show variable glucose consumption (and variable contrast agent uptake) inspite of their low aggressiveness [14]. The relation between tumor glucose consumption and prognosis has not yet been adequately studied for most rare tumor types, such as oligodendroglioma and ependymoma. Thus, [^{18}F]FDG-PET studies without histological diagnosis are of little clinical value.

To evaluate residual tumor after surgery, [^{18}F]FDG PET studies can be done already a few weeks postoperatively without artifacts due to wound healing, that invalidate contrast CT and MRI studies in that phase. [^{18}F]FDG uptake does not depend on blood-brain barrier disruption, and therefore adds information to malignancy estimates derived from contrast agent uptake. When MRI and CT cannot differentiate between recurrent tumor and radiation necrosis, both of which can exhibit contrast agent uptake, high glucose consumption (above that of normal gray matter) is rather specific (but not very sensitive) for recurrent tumor, whereas the clinical significance of intermediate (between normal gray and white matter) [^{18}F]FDG uptake is uncertain [15-17]. If [^{18}F]FDG uptake is higher than in the initial tumor, this may indicate further malignant degeneration [18]. It is important to note that [^{18}F]FDG PET must not be used to delineate or localize brain tumors. For interpretation, independent information on location and extent of pathological tissue (from CT, MRI or ^{11}C-methionine PET) is required.

Amino acids (^{11}C-methionine, ^{18}F-fluorotyrosine, ^{11}C-tyrosine) accumulate in most brain tumors [19-22] due to an increase of blood-to-tissue transport [23], including low grade gliomas that do not show uptake of contrast agents in CT or MRI and of Tl-201 in SPET [24]. They are therefore of particular value to determine location and extent of these tumors [25,26], and may therefore be used for planning of biopsy [27]. They also have a high sensitivity to detect recurrent or residual tumor. In clinical practice, delineation of tumors may occasionally be difficult because of variable background activity, and there are no clearly established objective thresholds to identify pathological accumulation. In a few cases, amino acid accumulation was absent in grade 2 astrocytomas. Accumulation of amino acids is not specific for brain tumors but may occur also in other acute brain lesions (e.g., recent ischemic infarcts with reperfusion). Yet, in chronic brain lesions it is probably useful as a tumor indicator. It is currently unknown whether differences in metabolism between the above mentioned amino acids lead to different behaviour for tumor imaging, and studies by Langen et al. [28] suggest that similar images can also be obtained with I-123-iodo-a-methyl-tyrosine and SPET. Monitoring treatment response is another potential clinical application for PET. A reduction of ^{11}C-methionine uptake after successful therapy was seen in pituitary adenomas [19] and in low-grade gliomas [29]. In lymphomas, which also show rapid response to radiation therapy in CT, PET was more sensitive to detect residual tumor [30]. Changes in [^{18}F]FDG uptake are less clear, and findings apparently depend on the time of scanning and type of therapy [31,32]

Cerebrovascular Disease (CVD)

Acute ischemic stroke is a leading cause of death and severe disability. In contrast to cardiac infarct, it does not hurt and therefore is often not experienced as an emergency by patients and physicians, leading to delay of treatment. PET significantly contributes to a better understanding of the pathophysiology of stroke and demonstrates the large interindividual variability of cerebral blood flow and metabolism in the first few hours after onset of ischemic stroke. Stroke treatment that takes into account this interindividual variability is likely to be much more successful than current approaches. Even moderate improvements will have enormous socio-economical consequences.

During the first few hours after ischemic stroke, CT and MRI with conventional imaging sequences do not show the extent and severity of ischemia, and during this phase, therapy leading to reperfusion, e.g. by thrombolysis, has the highest chance of saving part of the ischemic brain tissue. PET with O-15 labeled tracers (water, molecular oxygen, and carbon monoxide) to measure cerebral blood flow (CBF), tissue oxygen extraction and consumption can demonstrate the extent and severity of ischemia, and distinguish between irreversibly damaged and still viable tissue (see review by Heiss and Herholz) [33]. Currently, the complex logistics of PET usually prevent the use of PET for clinical diagnostics in this situation apart from research protocols. Ongoing research will show whether new MRI techniques (e.g. perfusion and diffusion weighted imaging) will be able to provide similar diagnostic information.

In patients with occlusion or high grade stenosis of brain vessels, the same technique can be used to quantify the degree of hemodynamic impairment [34,35]. This cannot be done by CBF measurement alone, because reductions of CBF can be secondary to reduced tissue metabolism, which may be caused by degenerative disease, past ischemia, or functional deactivation. In this frequent situation, any therapeutic attempts to increase blood blow probably do not yield any clinical benefit. Yet, misery perfusion [36], i.e. reduction of CBF below metabolic tissue needs as assessed by measurement of oxygen consumption, has been observed in a small proportion of patients with chronic CVD. In these patients, therapeutic improvement of CBF should contribute to stroke prevention, although adequate clinical studies have not yet been reported and preliminary results are controversial [37,38]. Measurements of the perfusion reserve by comparison of CBF at rest and during vasodilation with diamox (which can be done also with SPET and Xenon-CT) or measurements of increased capillary transit times (e.g., by dynamic CT and MRI after bolus application of contrast agents) have been shown to correlate to some degree with O-15 PET parameters [39,40]. Yet, the clinical diagnostic value of these techniques has not yet been compared systematically. In summary, PET provides detailed diagnostic information in chronic CVD, but its clinical impact relative to other techniques and with regard to therapy has not yet been fully evaluated.

Since [^{18}F]FDG-PET is a sensitive indicator of local brain dysfunction, it can also be used to localize cortical ischemic lesions with high sensitivity [41]. Small cortical ischemic infarcts may be hard to detect with CT and standard MRI techniques, because their signal is very similar to adjacent CSF. Areas with selective neuronal loss or functional deactivation can only be detected with functional imaging techniques like PET. Thus, impairment of rCMRGlu gives much better correlations with impairments of higher brain functions, e.g. aphasia [42,43], than imaging of brain infarcts with CT and MRI. In the subacute phase after acute ischemic stroke, rCMRGlu is of significant prognostic value. Global CMRGlu correlates with global outcome in terms of "activities of daily living (ADL)" scales [44], and regional CMRGlu correlates with outcome of specific functions, e.g. left temporo-parietal CMRGlu in the subacute phase correlates with recovery of language function after 1 year [45]. In principle, focal functional changes can also be identified with SPET using a commercially available flow tracer, e.g. Tc-99m-HMPAO, but, in absence of reliable absolute quantification, SPET data analysis requires a normal reference region, which is uncertain in patients with widespread vascular disease.

Degenerative Diseases

In the aging population of industrialized nations, the prevalence of Alzheimer's disease (AD) is still growing with large social and economical consequences. Diagnosis of dementia, including AD, usually can be made by clinical and neuropsychological examination. CT may be necessary to identify vascular lesions and to exclude rare conditions, such as frontal brain tumors or subdural hematoma. In a few cases, diagnosis may be difficult because of atypical presentation, predominant personality changes, concurrent depression, or early onset. In these cases diagnosis can be facilitated by [^{18}F]FDG PET, which exhibits typical regional metabolic changes in AD: bilateral reduction of rCMRGlu in temporo-parietal association cortex, and to a variable degree also of prefrontal association cortex, in contrast to relative preservation of rCMRGlu in primary visual and sensorimotor cortex, striatum and cerebellum (see review by Rapoport) [46]. By simple regional quantitative analysis, using a ratio of typically most affected through typically least affected regions, this pattern can be recognized objectively with comparable and reproducible results across laboratories [47].

Diagnosis of AD with [^{18}F]FDG PET is not always easy since limitations exist. As yet, PET cannot effectively detect metabolic changes in hippocampal structures, which are affected very early in the disease, when symptoms may be limited to memory impairment (which is not sufficient for clinical diagnosis). Thus, we do not know whether PET can improve early diagnosis of AD, since only unspecific findings (cortical asymmetries) have been described so far [48]. In very late-onset AD the typical pattern may be much less pronounced and unspecific global CMRGlu reduction may be predominant [49]. Yet, most data indicate that [^{18}F]FDG PET is very sensitive in early-onset AD, including familial cases. It can also be used to evaluate the effect of drugs [50,51]

Most other degenerative diseases can be recognized by regional reduction of CMRGlu in the affected brain structures, as listed in Table 2.

In contrast, Parkinsons's disease (PD), if not accompanied by dementia, does not lead to major changes of rCMRGlu, whereas PD with dementia shows metabolic changes very similar to AD [52]. Impairment of dopamine synthesis can be measured in the striatum by PET with ^{18}F-fluorodopa (^{18}F-Dopa) and correlates dopamine cell counts [53]. Because clinical symptoms appear only after loss of approx. Fifty % of

Table 2. Dementing and degenerative diseases with typical [^{18}F]FDG PET findings.

Disease	Brain areas with reduced CMRGlu
Alzheimer's	temporoparietal, variably frontal sparing: primary visual and sensorimotor cortex, striatum, cerebellum
Huntington's	striatum (caudate more than putamen)
Parkinson's with dementia	similar to Alzheimer's disease
Frontal lobe dementia (including Pick's)	frontal, in Pick's disease extending to anterior parts of temporal lobe
Vascular dementia	global or multifocal (incl. striatum and cerebellum)
Progressive supranuclear palsy	frontal and brainstem
Olivo-ponto-cerebellar atrophy	cerebellum, pons
Corticobasal ganglionic degeneration	lateral temporal and inferior parietal lobe, frontal operculum

Table 3. Clinical imaging of striatal dopamine synthesis and D_2 receptors in extrapyramidal disorders (after Brooks [57, 58]).

Disease	^{18}F-Dopa uptake	D_2 receptor density
Idiopathic parkinson's	reduced (with rostro-caudal gradient)*	normal or increased (upregulation)
Familial essential tremor	normal	?
Multisystem atrophy (striato-nigral degeneration and OPCA)	reduced (without rostro-caudal gradient)	normal or reduced
Pure autonomic failure	normal	?
Progressive supranuclear palsy	reduced (without rostro-caudal gradient)	normal or reduced
Wilson's	reduced	reduced
Corticobasal degeneration	reduced (without rostro-caudal gradient)	?
Dystonia	variable (reduced, normal, increased)	normal

?: insufficient data available.

*) rostro-caudal gradient: caudate less affected than putamen, and rostral parts of putamen less affected than caudal parts.

dopaminergic neurons, which corresponds to a similar reduction of ^{18}F-Dopa uptake, very early diagnosis and detection of preclinical disease in familial PD is possible with this technique [54-56]. If rare multisystem degenerations with parkinsonism are suspected clinically, measurement of receptor density with ^{11}C-raclopride or other D_2 receptor ligands is useful for differential diagnosis (see reviews by Brooks [57,58], and Table 3).

The clinical impact of PET in degenerative disease, in particular the possibility of early diagnosis, will increase when effective and specific drugs to stop or slow down disease progression become available. Since PET can measure disease progression objectively, it can help to perform clinical studies for testing drugs more effectively.

Conclusion

Clinical PET examinations should be done within scientific studies, at well equipped centers, and with highly experienced and specialized personnel to ensure high quality standards and an optimum gain of information (which depends on systematic comparisons of patients series) from this expensive technique. In some instances, PET may also provide a particular crucial item (e.g., the metabolic activity of a tumor, the degree of hemodynamic impairment, the extent of functional impairment) to complete diagnostic information and may thereby influence individual therapeutic decisions. To achieve that, PET requires very close cooperation and communication between the neurologist or neurosurgeon, who treats the patient, and the PET expert. Such cooperation is rarely seen in the setting of separate, independent departments. For clinical applications, the enormous amount of information that each PET examination of the brain yields is usually only used marginally by current methods of data processing and interpretation, and further research should therefore have priority over routine clinical applications. Yet, already now, clinical routine applications exist in differential diagnosis of degenerative brain diseases, treatment planning in brain tumors, to characterize hemodynamic and functional changes in cerebrovascular disease (as described above), and for diagnosis of focal epilepsy (as described in a separate chapter).

References

1. Russell DS, Rubinstein LJ. Pathology of tumours of the nervous system. 5th ed. London: Edward Arnold, 1989.
2. Pardo FS, Aronen HJ, Kennedy D, et al. Functional cerebral imaging in the evaluation and radiotherapeutic treatment planning of patients with malignant glioma. Int J Radiat Oncol Biol Phys 1994;30:663-669.
3. DiChiro G. Positron-emission-tomography using [F-18]-fluorodeoxyglucose in brain tumors - a powerful diagnostic and prognostic tool. Invest Radiol 1987;22:360-371.
4. Alavi JB, Alavi A, Chawluk J, et al. Positron emission tomography in patients with glioma - a predictor of prognosis. Cancer 1988;62:1074-1078.
5. Schifter T, Hoffman JM, Hanson MW, et al. Serial FDG-PET studies in the prediction of survival in patients with primary brain-tumors. J Comput Assist Tomogr 1993;17:509-516.
6. Hölzer T, Herholz K, Jeske J, Heiss D. FDG-PET as a prognostic indicator in radiochemotherapy of glioblastoma. J Comput Assist Tomogr 1993;17:681-687.
7. Shapiro WR. Low-grade gliomas - when to treat. Ann Neurol 1992;31:437-438.

8. Herholz K, Pietrzyk U, Voges J, et al. Correlation of glucose consumption and tumor-cell density in astrocytomas - a stereotaxic PET study. J Neurosurg 1993;79:853-858.
9. Goldman S, Levivier M, Bouquey D, et al. Correlation of glucose-metabolism and histopathology of gliomas using PET-guided stereotaxic biopsy. Neurology 1993;43:249-249.
10. Holthoff VA, Herholz K, Berthold F, et al. In-vivo metabolism of childhood posterior-fossa tumors and primitive neuroectodermal tumors before and after treatment. Cancer 1993;72:1394-1403.
11. DiChiro G, Hatazawa J, Katz DA, Rizzoli HV, DeMichele DJ. Glucose utilization by intracranial meningiomas as an index of tumor aggressivity and probability of recurrence: a PET study. Radiology 1987;164:521-6.
12. Cremerius U, Striepecke E, Henn W. et al. (18)FDG-PET in intracranial meningiomas versus grading, proliferation index, cellular density and cytogenetical analysis. Nuklearmedizin 1994;33:144-149.
13. DeSouza B, Brunetti A, Fulham MJ, et al. Pituitary microadenomas - a PET study. Radiology 1990;177:39-44.
14. Fulham MJ, Melisi JW, Nishimiya J, Dwyer AJ, DiChiro G. Neuroimaging of juvenile pilocytic astrocytomas - an enigma. Radiology 1993;189:221-225.
15. Doyle WK, Budinger TF, Valk PE, et al. Differentiation of cerebral radiation-necrosis from tumor recurrence by 18-FDG and Rb-82 PET. J Comput Assist Tomogr 1987;11:563-570.
16. Ogawa T, Kanno I, Shishido F, et al. Clinical-value of PET with F-18-fluorodeoxyglucose and l-methyl-C-11-methionine for diagnosis of recurrent brain-tumor and radiation-injury. Acta Radiol 1991;32:197-202.
17. Davis WK, Boyko OB, Hoffman JM, et al. [F-18]-2-fluoro-2- deoxyglucose positron emission tomography correlation of gadolinium-enhanced mr-imaging of central- nervous-system neoplasia. Am J Neuroradiol 1993;14:515-523.
18. Francavilla TL, Miletich RS, DiChiro G, Patronas NJ, Rizzoli HV, Wright DC. Positron emission tomography in the detection of malignant degeneration of low-grade-gliomas. Neurosurgery 1989;24:1-5.
19. Bergström M, Muhr C, Lundberg PO, Langstrom B. PET as a tool in the clinical-evaluation of pituitary adenomas. J Nucl Med 1991;32:610-615.
20. Bustany P, Chatel M, Delon JM, Darcel F, Sgouropoulos F, Syrota A. Brain-tumor protein-synthesis and histological-grades: a study by PET with C-11-l-methionine. J Neurooncol 1986;3:397-404.
21. Schober O, Duden C, Meyer GJ, Müller JA, Hundeshagen H. Non selective transport of C-11-methyl-l-methionine and d-methionine into malignant glioma. Eur J Nucl Med 1987;13:103-105.
22. Derlon JM, Bourdet C, Bustany P, et al. [C-11]-l-methionine uptake in gliomas. Neurosurgery 1989;25:720-728. [copy]
23. Wienhard K, Herholz K, Coenen HH, et al. Increased amino-acid-transport into brain-tumors measured by PET of l-(2-F-18)fluorotyrosine. J Nucl Med 1991;32:1338-1346.
24. Kameyama M, Shirane R, Itoh J, et al. The accumulation of C-11-methionine in cerebral glioma patients studied with PET. Acta Neurochir 1990;104:8-12.
25. Mosskin M, Ericson K, Hindmarsh T, Vonholst H, et al. Positron emission tomography compared with magnetic-resonance imaging and computed-tomography in supratentorial gliomas using multiple stereotactic biopsies as reference. Acta Radiol 1989;30:225-232.
26. Ogawa T, Shishido F, Kanno I, et al. Cerebral glioma - evaluation with methionine PET radiology 1993;186:45-53.
27. Go KG, Keuter EJW, Kamman RL, et al. Contribution of magnetic-resonance spectroscopic imaging and l-[1-C-11]tyrosine positron emission tomography to localization of cerebral gliomas for biopsy. Neurosurgery 1994;34:994-1002.

28. Langen KJ, Coenen HH, Roosen N, et al. Spect studies of brain-tumors with l-3-[I-123] iodo-alpha-methyl tyrosine - comparison with PET, 124imt and 1st clinical-results. J Nucl Med 1990;31:281-286.
29. Pietrzyk U, Herholz K, Würker M, et al. Effect of interstitial irradiation on glucose metabolism and methionine uptake in glioma patients. J Nucl Med 1994;35(suppl):235P.
30. Ogawa T, Kanno I, Hatazawa J, et al. Methionine PET for follow-up of radiation-therapy of primary lymphoma of the brain. Radiographics 1994;14:101-110.
31. Rozental JM, Levine RL, Nickles RJ. Changes in glucose uptake by malignant gliomas - preliminary-study of prognostic -significance. J Neurooncol 1991;10:75-83.
32. Dewitte O, Hildebrand J, Luxen A, Goldman S. Acute effect of carmustine on glucose-metabolism in brain and glioblastoma. Cancer 1994;74:2836-2842.
33. Heiss W.D., Herholz K. Assessment of pathophysiology of stroke by positron emission tomography. Eur J Nucl Med 1994;21:455-465.
34. Leblanc R, Yamamoto YL, Tyler JL, hakim A. Hemodynamic and metabolic effects of extracranial carotid disease. Can J Neurol Sci 1989;16:51-57.
35. Carpenter DA, Grubb RL, Powers WJ. Borderzone hemodynamics in cerebrovascular-disease. Neurology 1990;40:1587-1592.
36. Baron JC, Bousser MG, Rey A, Guillard A, Comar D, Castaigne P. Reversal of focal misery-perfusion-syndrome by extra-intracranial-arterial-bypass in hemodynamic cerebral ischemia - a case study with 15-O PET. Stroke 1981;12:454-459.
37. Samson Y, Baron JC. Pet studies in internal carotid occlusion patients: base-line hemodynamic and metabolic alterations: effects of surgical revascularization and induced arterial hypertension. In: Heiss WD, Pawlik G, Herholz K, Wienhard K, editors. Clinical Efficacy of Positron Emission Tomography, Dordrecht, Boston, Lancaster: M. Nijhoff Publ, 1987: 55.
38. Powers WJ, Grubb RL, Raichle ME. Clinical-results of extracranial-intracranial bypass-surgery in patients with hemodynamic cerebrovascular-disease. J Neurosurg 1989;70:61-67.
39. Herold S, Brown MM, Frackowiak RSJ, Mansfield AO, Thomas DJ, Marshall J. Assessment of cerebral hemodynamic reserve - correlation between PET parameters and CO2-reactivity measured by the intravenous Xe-133 injection technique J Neurol Neurosurg Psychiatry 1988;51:1045-1050.
40. Hirano T, Minematsu K, Hasegawa Y, Tanaka Y, Hayashida K, Yamaguchi T. Acetazolamide reactivity on I-123 imp single-photon emission computed-tomography in patients with major cerebral-artery occlusive disease - correlation with positron emission tomography parameters. J Cereb Blood Flow Metab 1994;14:763-770.
41. Heiss WD, Herholz K, Böcher-Schwarz HG, et al. PET, CT, and MR imaging in cerebrovascular disease. J Comput Assist Tomogr 1986;10:903-911.
42. Metter EJ. Neuroanatomy and physiology of aphasia: evidence from PET. Aphasiology 1987;1:3-33.
43. Karbe H, Herholz K, Szelies B, Pawlik G, Wienhard K, Heiss WD. Regional metabolic correlates of token-test results in cortical and subcortical left hemispheric infarction. Neurology 1989;39:1083-1088.
44. Heiss WD, Emunds HG, Herholz K. Cerebral glucose metabolism as a predictor of rehabilitation after ischemic stroke. Stroke 1993;24:1784-1788.
45. Karbe H, Kessler J, Herholz K, Fink GR, Heiss WD. Long-term prognosis of post-stroke aphasia studied with positron emission tomography. Arch Neurol 1995, in press.
46. Rapoport SI. Positron emission tomography in Alzheimer's disease in relation to disease pathogenesis - a critical-review. Cereb Brain Metab Rev 1991;3:297-335.

47. Herholz K, Perani D, Salmon E, FrancK G, Fazio F, Heiss W-D, Comar D. Comparability of FDG PET studies in probable Alzheimer's disease. J Nucl Med 1993;34:1460-1466.
48. Haxby JV, Grady CL, Koss E, et al. Longitudinal-study of cerebral metabolic asymmetries and associated neuropsychological patterns in early dementia of the Alzheimer type. Arch Neurol 1990;47:753-760.
49. Mielke R, Herholz K, Grond M, Kessler J, Heiss WD. Differences of regional cerebral glucose-metabolism between presenile and senile dementia of Alzheimer type. Neurobiol Aging 1992;13:93-98.
50. Heiss WD, Hebold I, Klinkhammer P, et al. Effect of piracetam on cerebral glucose-metabolism in Alzheimers-disease as measured by positron emission tomography. J Cereb Blood Flow Metab 1988;8:613-617.
51. Nordberg A. Effect of long-term treatment with tacrine (THA) in Alzheimer's disease as visualized by PET. Acta Neurol Scand 1993;88(suppl 149):62-65.
52. Kuhl D, Metter EJ, Riege WH. Patterns of lCmrglu determined in parkinson's disease by the FDG method. Ann Neurol 1984;15:419-424.
53. Snow BJ, Tooyama I, McGeer EG, et al. Human positron emission tomographic [F-18] fluorodopa studies correlate with dopamine cell counts and levels. Ann Neurol 1993;34:324-330.
54. Sawle GV, Wroe SJ, Lees AJ, Brooks DJ, Frackowiak RSJ. The identification of presymptomatic parkinsonism - clinical and F-18-dopa positron emission tomography studies in an irish kindred. Ann Neurol 1992;32:609-617.
55. Vingerhoets FJG, Snow BJ, Lee CS, Schulzer M, Mak E, Calne DB. Longitudinal fluorodopa positron emission tomographic studies of the evolution of idiopathic parkinsonism. Ann Neurol 1994;36:759-764.
56. Holthoff VA, Vieregge P, Kessler J, et al. Discordant twins with parkinsons-disease - positron emission tomography and early signs of impaired cognitive circuits. Ann Neurol 1994;36:176-182.
57. Brooks DJ. Positron emission tomographic studies of the subcortical degenerations and dystonia. Sem Neurol 1989;9:351-359.
58. Brooks DJ. PET studies on the early and differential diagnosis of Parkinson's disease. Neurology 1993;43(suppl 6):S6-S16.

11

POSITRON EMISSION TOMOGRAPHY IN PARTIAL EPILEPSY

Bernard Sadzot, René M.C. Debets, Eric Salmon, Cornelius W.M. van Veelen, Guy Delfiore, Alexander C. van Huffelen, George Franck

Uncontrolled partial epilepsy is an important medical problem. It can be surgically treated if the site of seizure onset, the epileptic focus, can be delimited and removed. Up to recently, accurate identification of the epileptogenic area relied solely upon sophisticated and time-consuming extra- and intracranial EEG recording techniques, even though EEG occasionnally may fail in providing the localization of the focus due to the rapid propagation of the electrical discharges.
Positron emission tomography (PET) allows to study non invasively and in vivo very specific physiological and biochemical variables including cerebral blood flow, oxygen and glucose metabolism. Radioligands are also available to image receptors and enzymes in the brain. Parameters that have been studied by PET in epileptic patients are summarized in Table 1.

Table 1. PET methods used in partial epilepsy

RADIOTRACER	VARIABLE ASSESSED
$C^{15}O_2$ / O_2	Blood Flow - Oxygen Metabolism
^{18}FDG	Glucose Metabolism
^{11}C-flumazenil	Benzodiazepine receptors
^{11}C-carfentanil	Mu-opiate receptors
^{11}C-diprenorphine	Mu, delta and kappa opiate receptors
3-^{18}F-acetylcyclofoxy	Mu, delta and kappa opiate receptors
^{11}C-deprenyl	Astrocytes - gliosis

The first tracer used in patients with partial epilepsy has been [^{18}F]fluorodeoxyglucose ([^{18}F]FDG) [1]; almost fifteen years later, it is still the most widely used. It is well established that interictal PET studies with [^{18}F]FDG demonstrate an area of glucose hypometabolism including the epileptic focus in the majority of epileptic patients. [^{18}F]FDG-PET and EEG are independent and complementary methods for the assessment of cerebral function. Consistency of EEG epileptic activity and hypometabolism within the same tissue volume leads to the probability that the hypometabolism is related to the presence of an epileptic focus and that the EEG abnormalities do not derive from the propagation of abnormal discharges that originate

R. Bares and G. Lucignani (eds.) Clinical PET, 103–113.

outside the hypometabolic volume. New biochemical tracers such as ^{11}C-flumazenil seem to demonstrate localized changes spatially more closely related to the epileptic focus.
Over the years, PET has gained a major role in the management of patients with partial epilepsy and has become a very useful, non invasive, confirmatory technique of functional disturbance associated with the epileptic focus. Single photon emission tomography (SPET) has followed. However, the assessment of cerebral function with SPET offers information that has not always been consistent with that obtained by PET, most likely because of the limited physical properties of SPET compared to PET, and to the features of the presently available SPET tracers. SPET offers unique advantages due to its wide availability and its flexibility for ictal studies in the work-up of epileptic patients.

Glucose Metabolism

It is now well established that in more than 70% of patients with partial epilepsy [^{18}F]FDG-PET shows a localized area of decreased brain glucose metabolism. PET however may be normal even in patients with well-defined EEG focus; at present, no patient should be rejected from an epilepsy surgery program on the sole basis of a normal PET study, but these patients may require more attention. Inversely, PET may show an area of decreased glucose utilization in patients with non localizing surface EEG or intracranial (IC-EEG) [2-10]. The hypometabolism may be regional or lobar and has usually a progressive demarcation from the normal cortex. It may also be more widespread and multilobar; in this case, the most hypometabolic lobe is the lobe of seizure onset [9]. The hypometabolic region may include an area with a more severe hypometabolism and a sharp demarcation from the adjacent, normal cortex: this condition often corresponds to a structural lesion. The site of ictal onset always lies within a demonstrated hypometabolic area. The hypometabolism is always on the same side of the brain as the epileptic focus although false lateralizations have very seldom been reported [4,10,11].
While glucose metabolism is a sensitive indicator, it is certainly not the ideal marker of the epileptic focus. Correlations with IC-EEG recordings have indeed indicated that the hypometabolism is usually wider than the epileptic focus. In temporal lobe epilepsy, the hypometabolism usually involves all the temporal cortex, while the epileptic focus is often confined to the mesial part of the temporal lobe [4,5,9]. In temporal (and in extratemporal) epilepsy, the metabolic data cannot be used as a guide for surgical resection. There are some indications that PET may allow to differentiate two TLE subgroups, a distinction that could have important therapeutic implications. In a recent study, Hajek et al. [12] found that patients with lateral (neocortical) temporal seizure origin had pronounced hypometabolism in the lateral temporal cortex but quite normal metabolic activity in the mesiobasal temporal lobe, while patients with mesiotemporal sclerosis had hypometabolism in both the mesial and the lateral cortex. For Henry et al. [13] however, mesiotemporal hypometabolism is observed not only in mesiotemporal epilepsy, but also in neocortical seizures, with or without a lesion. Mesiotemporal hypometabolism cannot be considered as a definitive evidence for the presence or absence of a histopathologic lesion in the hippocampus, nor for a limbic or a neocortical epileptic focus. More studies correlating IC-EEG recordings and metabolic patterns within the temporal lobe are required to clarify this very important issue.
There are few metabolic studies in partial epilepsies of neocortical origin. The regional patterns of interictal hypometabolism are much less characterized in these epilepsies than

in mesial TLE. [^{18}F]FDG-PET is more often normal; It may also show a circumscribed area of severe focal hypometabolism consistent with a structural lesion, as well as a lobar or multilobar hypometabolism [4,13-15].
A new generation of PET tomographs is now available on the market. They are characterized by a better temporal resolution (acquisition of time frames in the order of a second), which is an advantage for dynamic studies. They have also a better spatial sampling. Up to 30 slices can be acquired simultaneously. The entire brain volume can be scanned in a single acquisition. Studies can be resliced in the coronal plane, which is particularly useful when studying the temporal lobe, and more precisely of the amygdalo-hippocampal complex.

SPET vs PET

Single photon emission tomography (SPET) is based on another technology and on other isotopes. Because of the lower cost of the cameras, it is more widely available. Furthermore, the isotopes have a longer half-life, do not need to be produced by on-site cyclotron and are commercially available.
Apart from these advantages, SPET is characterized by lower performances in terms of both spatial and temporal resolution. It is also less sensitive. True isotope concentrations in a slice cannot be measured for technical reasons and absolute quantification cannot be obtained. Fewer tracers are available. They allow to measure blood flow ([^{99m}Tc]hexamethylene-propylene-amine-oxime, HMPAO; and [^{123}I]iodoamphetamine, IMP; and [^{99m}Tc]ethyl cysteinate dimer ECD) and more recently, some neuroreceptors ([^{123}I]-iomazenil, [^{123}I]-iododexetimide, [^{123}I]-IBZM). There is considerable interest in knowing whether SPECT performs as well as PET for patients with partial epilepsy in the setting of surgical treatment.
Interictal SPET studies in patients with temporal lobe epilepsy have provided highly variable results, with a sensitivity ranging from 80% to less than 50% [2,16-19]. Another source of concern is the frequency of false lateralizations, approximately 10%. When present, the degree of hypoperfusion is substantially lower than the asymmetry reported with PET. Some experienced workers in the field have even suggested that interictal SPET is unreliable [20]. Clearly, PET should be preferred to SPECT, whenever possible, particularly when such an important medical procedure as brain surgery is considered.
PET and SPECT have been carried out in the same epileptic patients and directly compared in two studies. Stefan et al. [21] have evaluated both imaging methods in 10 patients with TLE, 7 of whom had a unilateral EEG focus and a normal CT scan. All these 7 patients had an area of hypometabolism on PET whereas only 3 showed corresponding SPET abnormalities; in an additional patient, SPET lateralization differed from that obtained with PET and MRI. In another group of TLE patients with normal MRI, SPET was abnormal in 20% and PET in 80% while the sensitivity was similarly high (90 and 100 %, respectively) when MRI was abnormal [19]. The metabolic abnormalities not detected by SPET were always mild and restricted to the most anterior part of the lateral temporal cortex.
By contrast, peri-ictal SPET scans offer reliable localization in more than 70% of the cases. False lateralizations occur less frequently than with interictal scans. The radiopharmaceutical should be administered as rapidly as possible, ideally as soon as a seizure starts. Accurate documentation of the time of injection, as well as onset and termination of the seizure is vital for proper interpretation of these flow scans. Detailed studies have indeed identified rapid changes in blood flow distribution patterns from the

ictal to the post-ictal to late post-ictal states [17,18,20,22]. In rigourous and experienced hands, (peri-)ictal SPET seems more sensitive and reliable than interictal SPET for the presurgical localization of the epileptic focus. It is a useful tool, yielding informations complementary to that provided by ictal EEG, which cannot not always be interpreted.
Recently, reduced [^{123}I]iomazenil binding to benzodiazepine (BZ) receptors [23,24] and reduced [^{123}I]iododexetimide binding to acetylcholine receptors in the hippocampus [25] have been demonstrated by SPECT in patients with TLE. These studies remain preliminary and the interest of these tracers must be more extensively evaluated before recommanding widespread clinical application.

Blood Flow Studies With PET

Few blood flow studies have also been carried out interictally with PET in epileptic patients. They showed a reduction in blood flow in the temporal lobe with the epileptic focus [26,27]. [^{18}F]FDG-PET has however largely supplanted these flow studies that are now no longer carried out. Oxygen-15 emits positrons that are more energetic than those from fluorine-18 (1.72 versus 0.64 MeV); hence the positron range is longer for oxygen-15 than for fluorine-18 (8.2 versus 2.39 mm). Images obtained with oxygen-15 labeled molecules are more fuzzy, have a poorer resolution and a higher statistical noise than images obtained with fluorine-18 labeled compounds. Liederman et al. [28] investigated 28 patients with medically intractable partial epilepsy undergoing presurgical evaluation with PET scanning using both [^{18}F]FDG and $H_2{}^{15}O$. Among the 15 patients who had surgery or subdural electrodes, 3 patients showed falsely lateralizing $H_2{}^{15}O$-PET and 4 were normal. Only one [^{18}F]FDG-PET was normal and there was no discordant lateralization. [^{18}F]FDG-PET is more sensitive and specific for the lateralization and the localization of the epileptogenic area than methods using ^{15}O.

Receptor Studies With PET

With the appropriate radioligand, PET allows for imaging brain receptors. Highly specific maps (autoradiographies) of the major receptors in the brain (serotonin, dopamine, opiate, ...) have been obtained. Besides the interest of a better knowledge of the biochemistry of the epileptic focus, it rapidly appeared that brain receptor studies might also be of clinical interest. Like [^{18}F]FDG-PET, receptor imaging may help localize a "dysfunctional" area having some relationship with the epileptic focus.
PET has major advantages over in vitro biochemical analysis of pieces of temporal lobectomy from epileptic patients. It allows for in vivo measurements of these receptors, without disruption of the neuronal circuits or of their biochemical environment. It also allows for analysis of brain tissue adjacent to and remote from the epileptic focus ("internal controls").
Opiate receptors have first been studied in patients with complex partial seizures using PET and the selective and potent mu opiate agonist [^{11}C]carfentanil. Increased binding has been found in the lateral temporal cortex, at distance from the presumed epileptic focus, while binding was decreased in the amygdala region, probably reflecting tissue damage [29]. Interpretation of these findings is not straightforward, but in any case, this is the first indication in human that endogenous opioids may play a role in seizure disorders. No significant changes and no specific binding patterns were observed in

TLE patients studied with [^{11}C]diprenorphine [30] or with 3[^{18}F]acetylcyclofoxy [31]. These are less specific opiate ligands that bind with the same high affinity to mu, delta and kappa receptors. Opposite changes in mu and kappa receptors may explain these "negative" findings [30]. Specific ligands for delta and kappa receptors are being developped that may be used to answer this interesting question.

Benzodiazepine receptors are allosteric modulatory sites on the macromolecular complex that constitutes GABA receptors. Given that GABA is the major inhibitory neurotransmitter in the brain and that epilepsy is though to be the result of an imbalance between inhibitory and excitatory influences in the brain, it is not surprising that epileptologists have soon wanted to image the GABA-BZ receptor complex. There is to date no satisfactory PET ligand for GABA receptor itself, but the BZ receptor antagonist [^{11}C]flumazenil is an excellent PET ligand [32,33].

Savic et al. [34] were the first to report the in vivo demonstration of reduced BZ receptor density in the human brain. Several explanations are theoritically possible to explain this reduced binding: a) increased release of an endogenous ligand competing with the PET ligand for receptors that are normal in density and affinity; b) down regulation of receptors (in response to an increased release of endogenous ligand or as a part of the disease process); c) lower affinity of receptors for the PET ligand; d) loss of neurons expressing the receptor; e) in case of structural atrophy, decreased binding per unit of volume or apparent decrease due to volume averaging; f) any combination of the above.

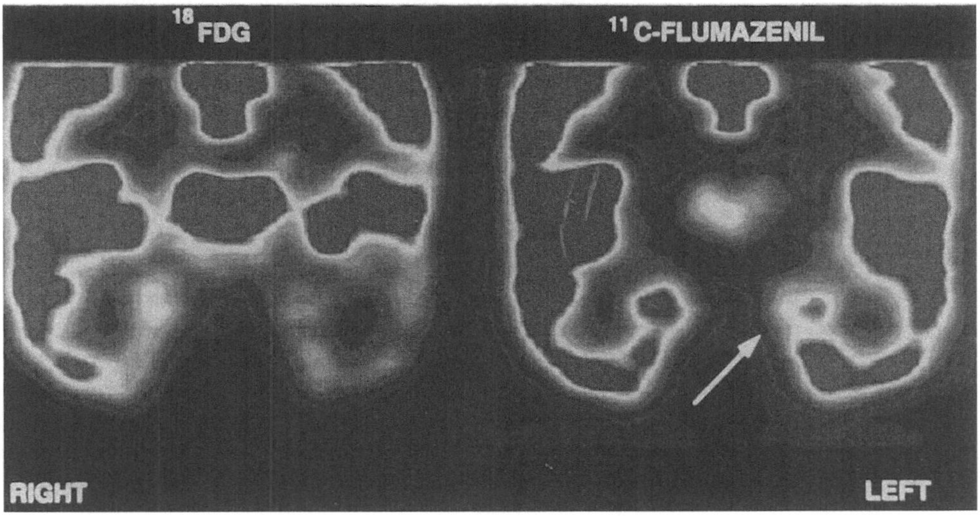

Figure 1. PET studies in a 26 year old female with complex partial seizures. Interictal and ictal surface EEG showed a left anterior temporal focus. MRI did not reveal signs of mesiotemporal sclerosis but a small area of increased signal intensity on T2 images in the left occipital white matter of questionable significance. PET showed a large area of glucose hypometabolism involving the left temporal lobe while the decrease in [^{11}C]flumazenil binding was restricted to the left hippocampus, as it can be seen on the 2 matched coronal planes. Based on the concordance between seizure semeiology, interictal and ictal EEG and PET, she underwent a temporal lobectomy without preliminary intracranial EEG recordings. The patient is seizure free 6 months after surgery.

The favourite hypothesis at this time is that [^{11}C]flumazenil is a marker of the neuronal loss associated with the epileptic focus. While these studies do not seem to bring new clues for the understanding of the pathophysiology of human epilepsy, they appear very promising from a clinical point of view.

Given the short half-life of carbon-11 and the rapid dissociation of the complex [^{11}C]flumazenil-receptor, it is possible to study during the same PET session [^{11}C]flumazenil binding and glucose consumption in the same individual. This protocol allows a direct comparison between these 2 biochemical parameters. Henry et al. [35] and ourselves [36] have shown that patients with TLE are characterized, on the epileptogenic side, by a reduction in [^{11}C]flumazenil binding limited to the mesial temporal region with little change in the lateral temporal cortex while glucose metabolism is reduced in both the mesial and the lateral temporal cortex, and sometimes in extratemporal areas. The decreased [^{11}C]flumazenil uptake in the hippocampus is particularly well demonstrated on the coronal planes. A representative example of these combined studies is shown Figure 1. This pattern has been observed in 90 % of a population of 30 consecutive patients candidate for epilepsy surgery referred to our PET center.

Both [^{11}C]flumazenil and [^{18}F]FDG are very sensitive markers in TLE. The area of decrease [^{11}C]flumazenil binding is spatially more limited and could have a closer relationship with the epileptic focus than the area of glucose hypometabolism. This question will be answered when more correlations with IC-EEG recordings will be available and when patients with extratemporal lobe epilepsy will have been investigated. In the end, [^{11}C]flumazenil could become the preferred PET tracer in patients with TLE, more especially as this ligand provides sharper images of the mesial and basal part of the temporal lobe than [^{18}F]FDG on coronal planes. A further advantage of this ligand is that the simple interpretation of the late uptake images is sufficient for clinical purposes. Compartmental modelling does not seem mandatory for a correct interpretation of the scans [37; personal experience].

PET may also be used to detect and highlight the gliosis associated with mesiotemporal sclerosis. Peripheral benzodiazepine receptors (PBZr) are associated in the brain with astrocytes and macrophages [38,39]. Rapid and marked increase in PBZr has been observed after various insults to the brain [40]. PK 11195, a ligand specific for PBZr, has been labelled with carbon-11. It has been used to image brain tumors in patients [41]. Increased [^{3}H]PK 11195 binding correlated with gliosis has been demonstrated by autoradiography in slices of hippocampus from patients with TLE [42]. [^{3}H]L-deprenyl binding was also increased. Deprenyl binds irreversibly and with high affinity to monoamine oxydase B [43]. In the brain, the B form is almost exclusively located extraneuronally, mainly on astrocytes [44]. [^{11}C]deprenyl and [^{11}C]deuterium-deprenyl have been used to label monoamine oxydase B in vivo with PET [45]. In a recent study, [^{11}C]deuterium-deprenyl uptake was increased throughout the temporal lobe harbouring a mesially situated epileptic focus in 6 patients with a unilateral focus [46]. This new PET method might be of limited interest however, given the high sensitivity of MRI for gliosis.

Quantification Of PET Studies

PET allows for precise regional measurements of radioactive tracers in slices of brain. Complex compartmental modelling methods have been designed to transform the regional radioactive concentrations into meaningful biological units (receptor affinity and density). The question is often raised whether quantification of PET studies is really necessary in clinical practice. It is not often carry out in radiologic procedures nor with SPECT. This question is important because simplification of the procedures leads to time saving and to lower cost.

The *regional* biochemical changes associated with *partial* epilepsy are easily detected by experienced eyes and quantification is not required for diagnosis purposes. If the PET method has been previously validated, which is important for a correct interpretation of the meaning of the procedure, plain scintigraphic images (and simple measurements: regional activity) are sufficient for clinical purposes; no sophisticated, elaborated kinetic compartmental modelling is required in routine. The procedure becomes much simpler. Regardless the clinical problem under study, the major advantage of visual interpretation is that the eyes integrate far more informations than those provided by few numbers in selected ROIs. In patients with partial epilepsy, visual interpretation of PET images may be superior to quantification for the detection of a localized change in a biological parameter, especially when one has just to compare one side of the brain to the other. Great attention should be paid however to factors affecting image quality: partial volume effect, counting statistics, color scale. Regional numbers may then come to support and complement the message of the parametric or the scintigraphic images, and to allow for interpopulation comparisons [47].

Conclusions

It is now admitted that in patients with temporal lobe seizures, an area of glucose hypometabolism is a reliable indicator of the localization of the epileptic focus in the concerned lobe. More precise localization of the epileptic focus in the affected temporal lobe (mesial versus lateral neocortical focus) could become possible with the newest PET camera and/or new tracers ([^{11}C]flumazenil). In patients with extratemporal epilepsy or with bilateral foci, PET may be less sensitive and more often normal. Further work with strict correlations between intracranial EEG and PET is required in these two categories of patients.

PET is one technique in many that can be used to localize the brain area constituting the epileptic focus. PET results should never be considered alone but should be integrated with other data to form a body of arguments towards a dysfunctioning brain region. In more and more centers, the congruence or concordance of clinical, electrophysiological, functional and anatomical informations towards a single brain region (i.e. the hippocampus), along with the absence of discordant data, is sufficient to embark on a surgical treatment [4,48]. The decision is thus more and more often based upon non invasive tests, without the need of preliminary intracranial EEG recordings. PET has progressively become a major criteria in non invasive presurgical evaluation protocols. It helps to select patients who could benefit more rapidly from standard anterior lobectomy. Elsewhere, it indicates patients who may require more attention, i.e. complementary intracranial investigations. It may also help to determine the type of evaluation (intracerebral or subdural electrodes) or to direct the placement of electrodes.

The development of new tracers, the refinement of image analysis and multimodality image co-registration (MRI and PET) will certainly further reinforce the place of PET in the non invasive evaluation of patients with partial epilepsy.

Acknowledgements

This work is supported by the Belgian Foundation for Scientific Research (FNRS) and The Queen Elisabeth Medical Foundation.

References

1. Kuhl, D.E., Engel, J. Jr, Phelps, M.E., Selin, C. Epileptic patterns of local cerebral metabolism and perfusion in humans determined by emission computed tomography of 18FDG and 13NH3. Ann. Neurol. 1980;8:348-360.
2. Abou-Khalil, B.W., Siegel, G.J., Sackellares, J.C., Gilman, S., Hichwa, R., Marshall, R. Positron emission tomography studies of cerebral glucose metabolism in chronic partial epilepsy. Ann. Neurol. 1987;22:480-486.
3. DeLaPena, R., Perlman, S.B., Levine, R., Kanner, A.M., Jones, J.J., Pyzalski, R., Nickles, R.J. PET scan findings in patients with temporal lobe epilepsy of mesial temporal origin. J. Nucl. Med. 1992;33:1014.
4. Engel, J., Jr, Henry, T.R., Risinger, M.W., Mazziotta, J.C., Sutherling, W.W., Levesque, M.F., Phelps, M.E. Presurgical evaluation for partial epilepsy: relative contribution of chronic depth-electrode recordings versus FDG-PET and scalp-sphenoidal ictal EEG. Neurology 1990;40:1670-1677.
5. Engel, J., Jr, Kuhl, D.E., Phelps, M.E., Crandall, P.H. Comparative localization of epileptic foci in partial epilepsy by PCT and EEG. Ann. Neurol. 1982a;12:529-537.
6. Engel, J., Jr, Kuhl, D.E., Phelps, M.E., Mazziotta, J.C. Interictal cerebral glucose metabolism in partial epilepsy and its relation to EEG changes. Ann. Neurol. 1982b;12:510-517.
7. Ryvlin, P., Cinotti, L., Froment, J.C., Le Bars, D., Landais, P., Chaze, M., Galy, G., Lavenne, F., Serra, J.P., Mauguière, F. Metabolic patterns associated with non-specific magnetic resonance imaging abnormalities in temporal lobe epilepsy. Brain 1991;114:2363-2383.
8. Sackellares, J.C., Siegel, G.J., Abou-Khalil, B.W., Hood, T.W., Gilman, S., McKeever, P.E., Hichwa, R.D., Hutchins, G.D. Differences between lateral and mesial temporal metabolism interictally in epilepsy of mesial temporal origin. Neurology 1990;40:1420-1426.
9. Sadzot, B., Debets, R.M., Maquet, P., van Veelen, C.W., Salmon, E., van Emde Boas, W., Velis, D.N., van Huffelen, A.C., Franck, G. Regional brain glucose metabolism in patients with complex partial seizures investigated by intracranial EEG. Epilepsy Res. 1992;12:121-129.
10. Theodore, W.H., Newmark, M.E., Sato, S., Brooks, R., Patronas, N., De La Paz, R., DiChiro, G., Kessler, R.M., Margolin, R., Manning, R.G., Channing, M., Porter, R.J. [18F]fluorodeoxyglucose positron emission tomography in refractory complex partial seizures. Ann. Neurol. 1983;14:429-437.
11. Swartz, B.E., Tomiyasu, U., Delgado-Escueta, A.V., Mandelkern, M., Khonsari, A. Neuroimaging in temporal lobe epilepsy: test sensitivity and relationships to pathology and post-operative outcome. Epilepsia 1992;33:624-634.
12. Hajek, M., Antonini, A., K.L. Leenders, Wieser, H.G. Mesiobasal versus lateral temporal lobe epilepsy: metabolic differences in the temporal lobe shown by interictal 18F-FDG positron emission tomography. Neurology 1993;43:79-86.
13. Henry, T.R., Sutherling, W.W., Engel, J. Jr, Risinger, M.W., Levesque, M.F., Mazziotta, J.C., Phelps, M.E. Interictal cerebral metabolism in partial epilepsies of neocortical origin. Epilepsy Res. 1991;10:174-182.
14. Radtke, R.A., Coleman, R.E., Hanson, M.W., Walczak, T.S., Lewis, D.V., McNamara, J.O. Positron emission tomography in extratemporal epilepsy. Neurology 1989;39 (Suppl. 1):301.

15. Swartz, B.E., Halgren, E., Delgado-Escueta, A.V., Mandelkern, M., Gee, M., Quinones, N., Blahd, W.H., Repchan, J. Neuroimaging in patients with seizures of probable frontal lobe origin. Epilepsia 1989;30:547-558.
16. Franceschi, M., Messa, C., Ferini-Strambi, L., Lucignani, G., Canal, N., Lenzi, G.L., Fazio, F. SPECT imaging of cerebral perfusion in patients with non-refractory temporal lobe epilepsy.. Acta Neurol. Scand. 1993;87:268-74.
17. Newton, M.R., Berkovic, S.F., Austin, M.C., Rowe, C.C., McKay, W.J., Bladin, P.F. Postictal switch in blood flow distribution and temporal lobe seizures.. J. Neurol. Neurosurg. Psychiat. 1992;55:891-894.
18. Rowe, C.C., Berkovic, S.F., Sia, S.T.B., Austin, M., McKay, W.J., Klanius, R.M., Bladin, P.F. Localization of epileptic foci with postictal single photon emission computed tomography. Ann. Neurol. 1989;26:660-668.
19. Ryvlin, Ph., Philippon, B., Cinotti, L., Froment, J.C., Le Bars, D., Maugiuère, F. Functional neuroimaging strategy in temporal lobe epilepsy: a comparative study of 18FDG-PET and 99mTc-HMPAO-SPECT. Ann. Neurol. 1992;31:650-656.
20. Rowe, C.C., Berkovic, S.F., Austin, M.C., Saling, M., Kalnins, R.M., McKay, W.J., Bladin, P.F. Visual and quantitative analysis of interictal SPECT with technetium-99m-HMPAO in temporal lobe epilepsy. J. Nucl. Med. 1991;32:1688-1991.
21. Stefan, H., Pawlik, G., Böcher-Schwarz, H.G., Biersack, H.J., Burr, W., Penin, H., Heiss, W.D. Functional and morphological abnormalities in temporal lobe epilepsy: a comparison of interictal and ictal EEG, CT, MRI, SPECT and PET. J. Neurol. 1987;234:377-384.
22. Duncan, R., Patterson, J., Roberts, R., Hadley, D.M., Bone I. Ictal/postictal SPECT in the pre-surgical localisation of complex partial seizures.. J. Neurol. Neurosurg. Psychiat. 1993;56:141-148.
23. Cordes, M., Henkes, H., Ferstl, F., Schmitz, B., Hierholzer, J., Schmidt, D., Felix, R. Evaluation of focal epilepsy: a SPECT scanning comparison of 123-I-iomazenil versus HM-PAO. Am. J. Neuroradiol. 1992;13:249-253.
24. van Huffelen, A.C., van Isselt, J.W., van Veelen, C.W., van Rijk, P.P., van Bentum, A.M., Dive, D., Maquet, P., Franck, G., Velis, D.N., van Emde Boas, W., Debets, R.M. Identification of the side of epileptic focus with 123I-Iomazenil SPECT. A comparison with 18FDG-PET and ictal EEG findings in patients with medically intractable complex partial seizures. Acta Neurochir. 1990;Supplementum 50:95-99.
25. Müller-Gärtner, H.W., Mayberg, H.S., Fisher, R.S., Lesser, R.P., Wilson, A.A., Ravert, H.T., Dannals, R.F., Wagner, H.N. Jr., Uematsu, S., Frost, J.J. Decreased hippocampal muscarinic cholinergic receptor binding measured by 123I-iododexetimide and single-photon emission computed tomography in epilepsy. Ann. Neurol. 1993;34:235-238.
26. Bernardi, S., Trimble, M.R., Frackowiak, R.S.J., Wise, R.J.S., Jones, T. An interictal study of partial epilepsy using positron emission tomography and the oxygen-15 inhalation technique. J. Neurol. Neurosurg. Psychiat. 1983;46:473-477.
27. Franck, G., Sadzot, B., Salmon, E., Depresseux, J.C., Grisar, T., Peters, J.M., Quaglia, L., Delfiore, G., Lamotte, D., Regional blood flow and metabolic rates in human focal epilepsy and status epilepticus. In: "Advances in Neurology: Basic Mechanisms of the Epilepsies", Vol 44, edited by A.V. Delgado-Escueta, Ward, A.A., Jr., D.M. Woodbury, and R.J. Porter. Raven Press, New York 1986;pp:935-948.
28. Leiderman, D.B., Balish, M., Sato, S., Kufta, C., Reeves, P., Gaillard, W.D., Theodore, W.H. Comparison of PET measurements of cerebral blood flow and glucose metabolism for the localization of human epileptic foci. Epilepsy Res. 1992;13:153-157.
29. Frost, J.J., Mayberg, H.S., Fisher, R.S., Douglass, K.H., Dannals, R.F., Links, J.M., Wilson, A.A., Ravert, H.T., Rosenbaum, A.E., Snyder, S.H., Wagner, H.N., Jr. Mu-opiate receptors measured by positron emission tomography are increased in temporal lobe epilepsy. Ann. Neurol. 1988;23:231-237.

30. Mayberg, H.S., Sadzot, B., Cidis Meltzer, C.C., Fisher, R.S., Lesser, R.P., Dannals, R.F., Lever, J.R., Wilson, A.A., Ravert, H. T., Wagner, H.N., Jr, Bryan, R.N., Cromwell, C.C., Frost, J.J. Quantification of mu and non-mu opiate receptors in temporal lobe epilepsy using positron emission tomography. Ann. Neurol. 1991;30:3-11.
31. Theodore, W.H., Carson, R.E., Andreasen, P., Zametkin, A., Blasberg, R., Leiderman, D.B., Rice, K., Newman, A., Channing, M., Dunn, B., Simpson, N., Herscovitch, P. PET imaging of opiate receptor binding in human epilepsy using [18F]cyclofoxy. Epilepsy Res. 1992;13:129-139.
32. Persson, A., Ehrin, E., Eriksson, L., Farde, L., Hedström, C-G., Litton, J.-E., Mindus, P., Sedvall, G. Imaging of [11C]-labelled Ro 15-1788 binding to benzodiazepine receptors in the human brain by positron emission tomography. J. Psychiat. Res. 1985;19:609-622.
33. Samson, Y., Hantraye, P., Baron, J.C., Soussaline, F., Comar, D., Mazière, M. Kinetics and displacement of [11C]Ro 15-1788, a benzodiazepine antagonist, studied in human brain in vivo by positron emission tomography. Eur. J. Pharmacol. 1985;110:247-251.
34. Savic, I., Persson, A., Roland, P., Pauli, S., Sedvall, G., Widen, L. In vivo demonstration of reduced benzodiazepine receptor binding in human epileptic foci. Lancet 1988;2:863-866.
35. Henry, T.R., Frey, K.A., Sackellares, J.C., Gilman, S., Koeppe, R.A., Brunberg, J.A., Ross, D.A., Berent, S., Young, A.B., Kuhl, D. In vivo cerebral metabolism and central benzodiazepine-receptor binding in temporal lobe epilepsy. Neurology 1993;43:1998-2006.
36. Sadzot, B., Debets, R.M., Delfiore, G., van Huffelen, C.W., van Veelen, A.C., Degueldre, C, Comar, D., Franck, G. Decrease of 11C-flumazenil binding is more localized than glucose hypometabolism in patients with TLE studied by PET. Neurology 1994;44 (Suppl. 2):A351-A352.
37. Savic, I., Ingvar, M., Stone-Elander, S. Comparison of [11C]flumazenil and [18F]FDG as PET markers of epileptic foci. J. Neurol. Neurosurg. Psychiat. 1993;56:615-621.
38. Syapin, P.J., Skolnick, P. Characterization of benzodiazepine binding sites in cultured cells of neuronal origin. J. Neurochem. 1979;32:1047-1051.
39. Zavala, F., Lenfant, M. Benzodiazepines and PK 11195 exert immunomodulating activities by binding on a specific receptor on macrophage . Ann. NY Acad. Sci. 1987;496:240-249.
40. Benavides, J., Cornu, P., Dennis, T., Dubois, A., Hauw, J.J., MacKenzie, Sazdovitch, V., Scatton, B., Imaging of human brain lesions with an omega 3 site radioligand. Ann. Neurol. 1988;24:708-712.
41. Junck, L., Olson, J.M., Ciliax, B.J., Koeppe, R.A., Watkins, G.L., Jewett, D.M., McKeever, P.E., Wieland, D.M., Kilbourn, M.R., Starosta-Rubinstein, S., Mancini, W.R., Kuhl, D.E., Greenberg, H.S., Young, A.B. PET imaging of human gliomas with ligands for the peripheral benzodiazepine binding site. Ann. Neurol. 1989;26:752-758.
42. Kumlien, E., Hilton-Brown, P., Spännare, B., Gillberg, P.G. In vitro quantitative autoradiography of [3H]-L-deprenyl and [3H]-PK 11195 binding sites in human epileptic hippocampus. Epilepsia 1992;33:610-617.
43. Knoll, J., Magyar, K. Some puzzling effects of monoamine oxydase inhibitors. Adv. Biochem. Psychopharmacol. 1972;5:393-408.
44. Nakamura, S., Kawamata, T., Akiguchi, I., Kameyama, M., Nakamura, N., Kimura, H. Expression of monoamine oxidase B activity in astrocytes of senile plaques. Acta Neuropathol. 1990;80:419-425.
45. Fowler, J.S., Wolf, A.P., MacGregor, R.R., et al. Mechanistic positron emission tomography studies: demonstration of a deuterium effect in the monoamine oxidase-catalyzed binding of 11C-L-deprenyl in living baboon brain. J. Neurochem. 1988;51:1524-1534.

46. Kumlien, E., Bergström, M., Lilja, A., Andersson, J., Szekeres, V., Westerberg, C-E., Westerberg, G., Antoni, G., Langström, B. Positron emission tomography with 11C-deuterium-deprenyl in temporal lobe epilepsy. Epilepsia 1994;In press:.
47. Sadzot, B., Debets, R.M.C., Maquet, P., Comar, C., Franck, G. PET data interpretation: visual inspection and semi-quantification/quantification. Acta Neurol. Scand. 1994;89:175-178.
48. Sperling, M.R., O'Connor, M.J., Saykin, A.J., Phillips, C.A., Morrel, M.J., Bridgman, P.A., French, J.A., Gonatas, N. A non invasive protocol for anterior temporal lobectomy. Neurology 1992;42:416-422.

Part Four:
Technical Requirements of a clinical PET-center

12

TECHNICAL REQUIREMENTS OF A CLINICAL PET CENTER: INSTRUMENTATION AND PERSONNEL

Christiaan Schiepers

Clinical PET has been a topic of major interest in recent years. The main reason is its unique ability to study physiological and biochemical processes in-vivo, and the association and characterization of disease states with altered blood flow, metabolism and/or receptor status. Initially, PET showed great potential in neurology, and after a shift of attention from neurological and psychiatric applications to cardiology in the eighties, we are now wittnessing an increasing interest in oncology. In the earlier sections, the application of PET in the main 3 clinical areas has been discussed.

The necessary equipment, i.e. cyclotron and automated chemistry, scanner and computers, archiving and hard copy devices, can be purchased from commercial companies. Several camera types allowing whole body scanning are available. Detector material and crystal size differ, directly affecting sensitivity, resolution and count rate. The reliability of scanners has improved significantly, the field of view extended, and industrial engineering has furnished easy to use equipment. Optimization of imaging protocols greatly reduced daily hands-on computer routines. As a consequence, the number of customers has increased, having a positive effect on the costs: prices came down, equipment down-time decreased and maintenance improved. Less expensive scanners are now available, some with a reduced number of detectors, and some small companies have been incorporated in strong multinationals. An overview of commercially available equipment in Europe in 1994 is given in Table 1.

Usually, PET systems produce 2-D images and a PET scan, in fact, consists of a stack of 2-D transaxial slices, varying in number between 7 and 61. 'This is accomplished by the septa in front of the detectors, limiting the number of lines of response (coincidence lines) to detectors in the same plane and their nearest neighbors in the z-direction. Modern systems have the capability to retract these septa for performing 3-D acquisitions. In 3-D mode, an increased number of detectors is 'in coincidence', encompassing the entire axial field-of-view. This increases the sensitivity of the camera by a factor 5-7. As an adverse effect, the scatter increases as well (up to 40%). The ECAT-ART and GE-QUEST (PENN-PET) do not have septa, they always acquire in 3-D mode. At this moment, 3-D reconstruction software is still under development. It is time consuming and not ready yet for clinical routine and will therefore not be considered here.

The following general steps can be distinguished in a PET study: 1) calibration scans, i.e. normalization, gain, blank; 2) rectilinear scan for positioning of the area of interest;

R. Bares and G. Lucignani (eds.) Clinical PET, 117–122.

Table 1. Overview of the presently available PET systems in Europe

Company	Model	Detector type	List price Million-ECU
Siemens	ECAT-EXACT 31-47-HR-ART	BGO	1.0 - 2.4
General Electric	ADVANCE	BGO	2.4
	QUEST	NaI	0.9
Positron Co	POSICAM HZ HZL HZL-R	BGO	1.7 - 2.5

BGO bismuth-germanate-oxide
NaI sodium iodide doped with thallium

The available scanning modes include: a)static - dynamic - gated; b) total body; c) 2D - 3D acquisition
All systems presently on the market are capable of performing the above mentioned scan-types. For brain and heart studies, adequate positioning is mandatory, especially for the smaller axial FOV cameras. Table positioning and remote control allow for flexible operations. Tables 2 and 3 give the typical sequence of operations in the 3 main PET examinations. Static studies are performed if the radio-activity distribution is at equilibrium or in a steady state, e.g. FDG metabolism. Dynamic studies are done if the time changes of the organ system of main interest are studied, e.g. blood flow and perfusion studies. Surveys of the body are typically performed in Onco-PET applications.
Four key steps may be distinguished in a PET study: 1) positioning, 2) transmission measurements with an external source, 3) injection of the tracer with a) simultaneous dynamic imaging and input function measurement (e.g. arterial blood sampling) or b) radiopharmaceutical uptake period, and 4) emission scanning. In general, dynamic acquisitions as well as attenuation correction are necessary to estimate absolute flow, metabolism or receptor density. In other words, a quantitative study is more demanding than a pure imaging study, which usually is sufficient for oncological total body surveys. On the other hand, semi-quantitative methods exist for static studies, e.g. Standardized Uptake Values (SUV) for brain and tumor imaging and monitoring of therapy response.
For high count rate studies, such as brain stimulation and organ perfusion, the dead time losses may become significant. NaI based systems (e.g. QUEST) suffer the most and are not well suited for this purpose. NaI based systems may be viewed upon as 'low count rate', ideally suited for OncoPET imaging. In fact, they are gamma cameras without 'an external collimator' but with coincidence electronics. The ECAT-ART with an incomplete detector ring and one revolution per two seconds, is a limited temporal sampling camera, adversely affecting the minimal frame duration or maximum frame rate that can be achieved. This may be insufficient for brain stimulation studies, but will perform well for routine perfusion imaging.

Table 2. Steps in a standard static and dynamic imaging studies. In a dynamic study the input function is a) sampled independently via arterial or arterialized blood or b) measured over a large area with an arterial blood pool, e.g. left atrium, left ventricle or aorta.

STATIC STUDY vs.	DYNAMIC / KINETIC STUDY
Rectilinear scan for positioning	Rectilinear scan for positioning
Stationary sequential bed positions	Stationary bed position
Transmission scan	Transmission scan
Delayed acquisition	Dynamic acquisition immediately
Quantification:	Quantification:
separately determined input function	Sampled - measured input function
standardized uptake values	Output Function, ROI analysis
uptake ratios	Kinetic Modeling

Table 3. In surveys of the body, a series of adjacent bed positions is acquired to encompass the entire are of interest. Obviously, the radioactivity distribution needs to be in a 'steady state'.

TOTAL BODY SURVEY	
Multiple bed positions	
Transmission scan of limited area	
Uptake interval after tracer administration	
Set of short static acquisitions	
Quantification:	standardized uptake values
	uptake ratios

Typical technical and performance values as listed are given in Table 4 for the various systems available in Europe. In general, the resolution of state-of-the-art cameras is in the order of 5 mm, which in clinical practice amounts to 8-10 mm due to filtering and patient or organ motions. Nowadays, rotating rod or pin sources are installed to acquire transmission scans instead of ring sources. This supplies a higher positron flux, and permits to perform transmission measurements after the radiopharmaceutical has been injected, i.e. after the emission scan. In this way the patient can be positioned later in the scanner, after the uptake period of tracer, leading to shorter scanner times, fewer motion artifacts and enhanced patient throughput. All scanners are equipped with modern computer platforms (SUN, HP, Digital workstations) that handle acquisition, reconstruction, image display and some kind of database management. In addition, a variety of hard copy devices is offered, e.g. film, laser printers (color - B/W), slides.
Most vendors have packages for 2D and 3D display, oblique re-orientation, and total body mode presentation. Software for measured as well as calculated attenuation

Most vendors have packages for 2D and 3D display, oblique re-orientation, and total body mode presentation. Software for measured as well as calculated attenuation correction is supplied by all manufacturers. More sophisticated models are left to the researchers. Regions and curves operation is usually available. Simple (semi)-quantitative software for SUV and Patlak graphical analysis is not always present. Parametric mapping, which is standard in the single photon applications for cardiac studies, is in general not implemented by PET software engineering. Concerning modeling, a static FDG model for the calculation of glucose utilization, and a model to compute absolute myocardial perfusion is sometimes available. Development of other kinetic models is left to the customer.

Table 4. Technical performance of the various positron cameras

Company/Type	Opening (cm)	Slices (mm)	axFOV (cm)	Sensitivity (Kps/mCi/ml)	Resolution (mm)
Siemens/ECAT	60	31-61	108-162	200-240	4.2-6.8
GE/ADVANCE	55	35	152	210	4.2
QUEST	50	128	250	350	5.5
Positron/POSICAM	53	45-61	125-166	200-260	5.8

Opening: effective size of camera aperture to pass patient
axFOV: axial Field-of-View

In the typical clinical setting an on-site cyclotron plus (automated) radiochemistry is not required. FDG, the work horse of PET, could be dispensed by a nearby radiopharmacy (satellite concept). Various companies sell cyclotrons or chemistry equipment, as do major vendors. For a more detailed discussion the reader is referred to the radiopharmacy presentation. The cost of a complete laboratory including a small cyclotron may vary between 750 and 2050 kECU. All companies offer a complete set for the generation of C-11, N-13, O-15 and F-18 and the frequently used radiopharmaceuticals water, oxygen, carbon-monoxide and dioxide, ammonia, FDG. Presently available systems in Europe are summarized in Table 5.

Table 5. Cyclotrons available in Europe. Most manufacturers sell automated chemistry for routine production of FDG, ammonia, oxygen, water etc.

Company/Type	Proton MeV	Target Positions	Extraction Beams
Siemens/RDS-112	11	4	2
GE/PET-trace	16.5	6	2
Oxford/Clinitron	12	7	1
IBA/Cyclone	3-10-18	1-8-8	1-2-2

The support required, in general, to operate a PET system is given in Table 6. With an estimated cost (in thousands of ECU) of 280 for personnel, 300 for maintenance, 100 for supplies, 300 for the building, and 600 for annual annuity the fixed operational costs for 1 year amount to 1580 . A projected number of 800 studies/year (i.e. 20/week) would fix the price to about 2000 ECU/study. The translation of the support into personnel depends on several factors. The above estimation (Table 6) may therefore vary considerably. For the operation of a PET facility, external services can be contracted. This is routinely done for maintenance, both for cyclotron/radiopharmacy and camera/computer. If the radiopharmaceuticals are dispensed by an external company or PET center, obviously, this part of the costs can be decreased and chemistry personnel costs omitted. This external delivery is at the expense of flexibility and number of tracers available. F-18 FDG can be delivered over distances that take 1-2 hours transportation. For the other radiopharmaceuticals this is virtually impossible. Generator nuclides (Rb-82, Cu-62) may be attractive alternatives for N-13.

Table 6. Estimated fixed and variable costs of a clinical PET center.

Personnel		#	Time	Total Costs
Mechanics and maintenance		engineer	service contract	
Physics and software		physicist	full	50 k
Cyclotron and radiopharmacy		pharmacist	part	50 k
		technologist	full	30 k
Medical		physician	part	90 k
		technologist	full	30 k
Administrative		clerk	part	30 k
Total				280 k
Equipment	Camera / Computers			1.1 - 2.7 M
	Cyclotron/ Chemistry			0.8 - 2.0 M
	Maintenance			10% / yr
Housing	building			100 k
	cleaning			
	supplies: medical, chemical, energy			200 k /yr

Personnel requirements in time and costs in k ECU.
Costs for equipment in M ECU.
Maintenance, supplies are expressed as k ECU / year.

Mandatory personnel for the facility are a physicist for technical support, calibration, and software; a technologist to perform the scans; a physician for medical interventions and reading; and administrative services for scheduling, typework, and billing. This scenario assumes a full maintenance contract to repair the scanner within 24 hours, which in general amounts to about 10% of the equipment price per year. The lower limit cost of personnel is estimated at 280 kECU. An additional radiopharmacist and technologist for equipment and personnel to operate a clinical PET facility may vary between (in million ECU): 1.6 - 5 for the initial purchase, 0.2 - 0.5 for maintenance per year, 0.25 - 0.35 personnel costs per year, about 0.3 for housing, heating, cleaning, etc. The costs may be diminished significantly by assigning duties to already available personnel in Nuclear Medicine, Radiology, e.g. physicians, secretaries, receptionist, and by reassignment of available rooms to the PET system. The price of room shielding for the higher photon energies is usually not prohibitive. However, this may be a significant factor for cyclotron and radiopharmacy. By sharing personnel, re-allocation of duties and space, expansion of an already available service, Clinical PET is feasible, even in these less favorable economic times. The functional information provided by PET in the fields of neurology, cardiology, psichiatry and oncology is unique and has a direct impact on patient management by aiding in diagnosis, prognosis, and monitoring the response to therapy.

References

1. Siemens. Technical DATA on ECAT EXACT systems.
2. 1994 ECAT users meeting book, Louvain-la-Neuve, Belgium.
3. General Electric. Product data form on ADVANCE, QUEST and PETTRACE.
4. Positron Corporation. Systems and options specifications.
5. Ion Beam Application. PET compound production systems.
6. Saha GB, MacIntyre WJ, Go RT. Cyclotrons and PET radiopharmaceuticals for clinical imaging. Sem Nucl Med 1992;22:150-161.
7. Koeppe RA, Hutchins GD. Instrumentation for PET: tomographs and data processing and display systems. Sem Nucl Med 1992;22:162-181.

13

TECHNICAL REQUIREMENTS OF A CLINICAL PET CENTER: DATA ACQUISITION AND PROCESSING

Stefan P. Müller

An objective assessment of the demands for data acquisition and processing capabilities and of the changes associated with the evolution of PET from a pure research tool into a clinical modality is almost impossible. Clinical PET is still an emerging technique which is not yet widely available for patient care. The future impact of PET on patient management in various diagnostic entities can only be projected today. The application of PET, however, is the major determinant for the technical capabilities required for the hard and software. Unfortunately, the technical evolution of PET hardware and software itself may change the practice of clinical PET in the future; e.g., there were no relevant clinical application of dynamic studies with single slice scanners, however, the availability of modern volume imagers, which can acquire dynamic data over a clinically useful field-of-view, may make quantitative dynamic approaches interesting for selected clinical questions. A validation, however, has to await the more widespread availability of these systems in the clinical PET community. Since PET systems are long-term investments, great care has to be exercised not to lock the clinical user of tomorrow into limitations imposed by the hardware which are conceived from the limited perspective of clinical PET today. Although it may be worthwhile to investigate these questions in a more rigorous way, this exceeds the scope of this article. Therefore, this paper will present a subjective view of several issues of data acquisition and processing in PET which stems from our own experience of starting up and running a PET center with basic and clinical research as well as patient care.

The transition of PET from a research tool to a clinical modality has changed the requirements imposed on hardware as well as software design. Formerly, strong emphasis was placed on the flexible implementation of research protocols which necessitate absolute quantitative capabilities. Only a limited number of these studies per day were performed in a typical research environment. The emerging clinical requirements emphasize imaging studies of extended areas of the body, however, the demands on quantitation are typically limited (e.g. standardized uptake values), but high patient throughput is of utmost importance to ensure cost effective operation.

At the same time the technical sophistication of PET users has undergone a transition. Unlike the typical research staff with ample technical expertise, some of the current clinical users are naive about the underlying physical, technical, and physiological aspects of a PET study. This mandates software which is simple to use and provides safeguards against operator errors.

If PET is to succeed as a clinical modality, and, at the same time, remain a scientific frontier of innovation in nuclear medicine, these two divergent requirements have to be

R. Bares and G. Lucignani (eds.) Clinical PET, 123–130.

reconciled in the design of hardware and software for future generations of PET systems. A main reservation against the success of clinical PET is the high cost per study. Improved patient throughput is a major determinant to dispel this prejudice. Several hardware and software factors determine the number of patients which can be studied in a given time.

Attenuation Correction

One of the major problems with current generation scanners available in the field is the necessity to perform the transmission scan for the attenuation correction before any tracer is administered to the patient. A measured attenuation correction is necessary to obtain quantitatively accurate images, especially in studies involving areas of inhomogenous attenuation or complicated body contours (e.g. in the chest, or the transition from the neck to the thorax). It is imperative that the position of the patient is not changed between the transmission scan and the emission scan to avoid grave artifacts which may mimic lesions and severely deteriorate the diagnostic accuracy of PET. E.g. in static FDG imaging, where a delay between the injection of the radiopharmaceutical and the acquisition of the emission data is necessary, the patient has to spend this waiting period in the scanner, blocking its use for other applications, while no data are being acquired. There are two approaches to eliminate this inefficient use of the scanner. First, using masked rod sources, it may be possible to perform the attenuation scan after, or, for low-count-rate studies, even simultaneously with the emission scan. An additional benefit of this approach is that artifacts due to involuntary positional shifts of the patient on the scanner bed between attenuation and transmission measurement can be avoided. A second approach may involve exact repositioning of the patient between attenuation and emission measurements, conceivably using software realignment of the data sets. Potential and limitation of both approaches has to be validated further before they can be recommended for a clinical routine setting.

PET has the potential for quantitative measurements. Scanners targeted for the clinical imaging market today should not give up this capability, since a PET scanner is a long-term investment, and the ultimate role of clinical PET is not yet defined. Therefore, accurate attenuation correction software should be available for all modes of scanner operation, including whole body acquisition. The software should allow the user to perform attenuation correction based on transmission scans, as well as calculated corrections based on body contours and segmented images with assigned attenuation coefficients.

Axial Field-of-View

The second major requirement is a sufficiently large axial field-of-view to cover the area of interest in the body. If the FOV is smaller than the region necessary to answer a given clinical question, multiple attenuation and emission scans in different axial positions must be acquired. If the transmission scan must be acquired before tracer administration, low patient throughput will result. In addition, the necessity for multiple axial scans precludes dynamic scans to investigate the kinetics of non-stationary radiopharmaceuticals. Considering the emerging clinical role of PET in oncology, which often demands whole-body imaging, any increase in the axial extent of the field-of-view is highly welcome. Regardless of the imaging task at hand, a large axial FOV simplifies patient positioning and therefore, helps to reduce the setup time and improves patient throughput.

3D-Acquisition

An additional important benefit of an extended axial field-of-view is the increased sensitivity when the interplane septa are removed and all lines of response are used in conjunction with three-dimensional reconstruction. This improvement in sensitivity can be translated to reduced imaging times for the same statistical quality of image data compared to a conventional PET scanner with septa and 2D reconstruction. An undesirable side effect of 3D acquisition, however, is the increased number of scattered photons which contribute to the image. As yet there is no consensus about optimal scatter correction, a fact which limits valid quantitative applications of 3D imaging to technically sophisticated users.

Data Handling

The transition to larger axial fields-of-view and especially to 3D acquisition leads to a significant increase in the size of the sinogram data by up to 2 orders of magnitude. This requires more efficient means for data handling and archiving than those currently available. Under practical considerations an on-line storage capacity for all raw and image data from at least 2 working days should be available. The management of the large amount of data would be facilitated by a searcheable patient database for the archival and retrieval of raw data, as well as processed image datasets. This tool should also ensure that complete datasets are archived (e.g., that for all sinogram data there is always the appropriate normalization scan available). In addition, all additional data should be integrated directly with the file structure, e.g. gating information or external blood data. To compare the PET data with other imaging modalities, file import and export facilities for standard formats (Interfile, ACR/NEMA) should be provided.

Quality Assurance

In order to free scanner time for patient studies, all procedures for quality assurance should be automated to run overnight. A report in a format readable for trained scanner operators, as opposed to physicists with research interest in PET hardware, should be available every morning.

Patient Positioning Aides

A contributing factor for improved patient throughput is easy patient positioning. Software positioning aides, maybe even in the form of a "persistence scope" display for an anterior and lateral planar projection in transmission as well as emission mode, would shorten the time for patient positioning, especially if the scanner has a small FOV relative to the volume of interest in the patient. Likewise, the total counts within the field-of-view should be available in a graphic display before the initiation as well as during the acquisition of the scan.

Predefined Protocols

Similarly to established imaging modalities with high patient throughput, e.g., CT or MRI, a basic set of predefined acquisition protocols should be provided by the manufacturer; of course, modification and extension with additional protocols by the user must be possible. These protocols should cover parameters of acquisition, processing, and patient documentation.

Reconstruction and Filtering

With the availability of larger axial data sets PET has evolved from being a slice-by-slice to a volumetric imaging modality. This must be reflected in the data reconstruction and filtering package, where flexible 3-dimensional filtering and image processing functions should be available. It might be helpful for clinical PET sites if the reconstruction and filtering options could be assigned from a clinical imaging protocol.
We believe that iterative reconstruction algorithms should be integrated into current PET reconstruction packages. We acknowledge that many questions regarding theoretical as well as implementation issues have not been addressed conclusively in the scientific community, such as the fitting criteria (e.g., least squares, maximum-likelihood, Bayesian), the regularization and stopping rule (e.g., fixed number of iterations vs. figure-of-merit), or the minimization algorithm (e.g., the expectation maximization algorithm and its derivatives or algebraic reconstruction techniques), and other questions. Nevertheless, there is clear indication that iterative reconstruction algorithms may perform better than filtered backprojection when areas of low activity concentrations must be evaluated in the presence of structures with high activity concentration within the same slice. This type of imaging tasks occurs frequently in oncological PET imaging (e.g., when FDG activity is excreted with high concentration in structures of the urinary tract); other situations are, e.g. catheters in the slice.

3D Visualization

The evolution of PET into a volumetric imaging method demands new paradigms for the data analysis and display software. In contrast to the small number of slices obtained with previous generation PET scanners, a large volumetric dataset with up to hundreds of slices for whole body scans may be acquired with the hardware available today, rendering a slice-by-slice evaluation obsolete. Display tools for 3D data should help to exploit the 3-dimensional relationship between structures of interest in the data and integrate them in a suitable way for the most powerful image processing and decision making device, the human brain. Further research into an objective comparative assessment of 3D display modalities for relevant imaging tasks should be encouraged.
The clinician may be aided by familiar displays. In nuclear medicine, projection images onto orthogonal planes are familiar to all practitioners. These should be available as static as well as rotating projection displays. It should be recognized, however, that all projection techniques (e.g., the maximum of the projection ray, the integral along the projection, or depth weighted schemes) are not equally suitable for various lesion detection tasks, especially for cold lesions.
Another familiar display modality for volumetric image data stems from B-mode ultrasound. Current computer hardware makes possible a similar real time dynamic reslicing tool, however, a new input device, which provides more degrees of freedom

than a mouse or a joystick, would be necessary to give the true "look and feel". This approach provides slices under arbitrary angles and allows to appreciate the full threedimensional topographic relationship among structures of interest.
For cardiac studies special formats for display and analysis (e.g., quantitative bulls eye plots of the myocardium) have been available in conventional nuclear medicine; these approaches lend themselves to cardiac 3D PET data as well. If the software is flexible enough, similar polar representations of organ surfaces may be applied to other organs (e.g., to the cerebral cortex).

Image Registration

More and more applications in clinical PET benefit from a direct correlation of the functional PET information with morphological data from, e.g., CT or MRI, or, e.g., from SPECT studies. The scanner software should provide a simple interface to import data from these modalities. Moreover, although the issues of optimal image registration and validation of its accuracy are not answered, we feel that registration tools for the realignment of PET data with morphological data, based on internal and external fiducial markers as well as surface matching techniques, should be available today. No automatic registration package can be expected to yield good results under all conceivable circumstances; therefore, a flexible visualization package must be available which would allow the user to assess quickly the quality of the coregistration achieved by the algorithm and perform necessary corrections manually. Furthermore, the software should simplify the association of findings in a synoptic display of individual resliced PET images, projection views, and displays from other modalities (e.g., with superimposed markers).

Dynamic Data

From the beginning, PET has included the temporal domain of tracer accumulation. Even in the age of clinical PET as a predominantly static imaging modality, dynamic data acquisition and processing capabilities must not be sacrificed. One should not forget that the larger axial FOV of modern day scanners allows us to acquire kinetic data over large enough areas in the body to be of clinical interest. Much additional quantitative information may be gained from regional tracer kinetics once tracer kinetic analysis methods mature to become routine applications. Therefore, adaptable data analysis software for dynamic data, including flexible frame manipulations, is required. Likewise, a versatile plotting tool for visualizing and analyzing time-activity-curves should be integrated in the data analysis package.

Modeling

Tracer kinetic modeling is largely a research tool today, yet it has been demonstrated that the diagnostic quality of modeled parametric images can be far superior to simple static maps of tracer uptake (e.g., images of the metabolic rate of FDG for the detection of liver tumors). In cardiac imaging as well, absolute maps of flow and metabolism may enhance the diagnostic potential of PET. It is time to start integrating simple modeling tools into the clinical software package (e.g., FDG metabolism, flow (NH3, H2O), and a tool for Gjedde-Patlak analysis). In the context of clinical applications the generation of parametric images should be emphasized over ROI-based modeling. Any modeling package should be based on a general extensible framework which facilitates the addition of new models once they have been clinically validated. Input function data, either generated from ROI's or imported from external counting systems, should be fully integrated in the file formats. We recognize that there are potentially grave risks in providing a clinical user, inexperienced with tracer kinetic principles, with modeling tools, however, ten years back, emission computed tomography itself - either SPECT or PET - was not in the realm of the average user but rather restricted to few experts with scientific expertise in the field. Education and legally mandated quality control measures, which are reflected in current SPECT software packages, brought this methodology to the clinical routine; a similar evolution should be envisioned for tracer kinetic modeling. At least initially, modeling tools could be locked into "approved" predefined protocols and the software might check the radiopharmaceutical, as entered in the database, and the acquisition parameters for plausibility. Finally, warnings should be displayed if the errors for the modeled parameters or the goodness-of-fit, calculated from the raw data, exceed predefined limits.

ROI Manipulation

In many instances, a quantitative or semiquantitative assessment of tracer uptake or derived parameters in a structure of interest must be performed. The software tool for the evaluation of these regions-of-interest should be applicable to all image displays; likewise, it should be possible to display and document the result of a ROI evaluation - with appropriate units - directly in the image from which is was derived. The 3D datasets from modern scanners provide the opportunity to improve substantially the precision of ROI-based measurements, simply by using the available information in all appropriate slices - a potential currently not used adequately. A ROI tool should be integrated with the 3D visualization software to accommodate the easy manual placement of ROI's in 3D. In addition, automatic ROI generation, based on simple local thresholding as well as more advanced image segmentation techniques, is necessary. The availability of an input device with more degrees-of-freedom than a mouse may greatly simplify the task of placing or modifying 3D ROI's in a volumetric dataset.

General Software Design and Documentation

The paradigm change for PET from a pure research instrument to a clinical tool mandates a different general approach to software design, documentation, and user training. The typical research user of the past usually had a sound background in the physical and technical foundations of PET, as well as experience with computer operation and system management, but this cannot be expected from a clinical user.

An improvement of the software stability is of utmost importance. Considering the increasing time required for processing or transferring the large datasets it is essential that all functions (i.e., data acquisition, data processing, and data archival) can be performed concurrently without jeopardizing, e.g., a running acquisition on the scanner.

The software should turn into a guide in addition to being a mere tool for scanner operation. A graphical user interface for scanner operation, data analysis, and routine system management is highly desirable; emphasis should be put on a consistent use of menus, buttons, command keys, etc. across all modules of the software. There should be warning messages for implausible or illegal operations (e.g., selecting a long scan duration for 15O-labeled radiopharmaceuticals, discrepant bed positions between transmission and emission scans, etc.). The acquisition of normalization and calibration data especially should be extensively safeguarded by the software, since errors during these crucial steps invalidate the results from a large number of scans and are often difficult to notice, especially for technically less experienced personnel. All system messages or warnings should be easily understandable in plain text, or even supplemented with pictorial aides, rather than cryptic abbreviations, acronyms, or error numbers. In addition. an extensive integrated on-line help facility should be available for all functions and system messages. Nevertheless, the software should be easily extensible and provide means to override these safeguards for novel research applications by technically sophisticated users.

The best documentation cannot compensate for the lack of a thorough training of new users. The specific needs of technical support personnel and clinicians should be addressed appropriately. Nevertheless, the documentation should be improved. For clinical users in particular there is a strong need for a tutorial style guide which covers operation and trouble shooting from basic to more advanced applications. The chapters could be set up to start with a short introduction, which covers underlying basic principles, followed by a step-by-step description of the procedures for operation. The section on attenuation correction, e.g., might start with a brief discussion of the consequences of attenuation on the image and derived quantitative parameters, approaches for attenuation correction, and their suitability for various situations; caveats about the dangers of inappropriate usage of available options should be covered here as well.

This tutorial guide does not obviate the need for a detailed reference manual, where sound background information should be provided about the underlying operational concepts of all functions provided by the system. This manual should also give exact mathematical definitions for system functions (e.g., the dead time correction or scatter correction algorithms) as well as for data analysis procedures (e.g., for quantities derived from ROI's or by tracer kinetic modeling). In addition, a detailed description of the file header information should be provided to fulfill the needs of the research community.

Finally, a keyword cross reference should be available to find quickly in-depth information to any given problem or topic of interest. Obviously a consistent use of units, terminology, and notation should be applied throughout the entire documentation, as well as in the on-line help system.

Patient Documentation

Documentation of the results of a clinical PET study is far more than a question of esthetic preference; it is a legal requirement. Note that the documented study must suffice as evidence, e.g., in a malpractice suit. The possible legal relevance of the documented images requires high-quality black & white or color output devices. Whereas the documentation of 10 or 20 individual slices was practical for older PET scanners, different approaches must be found for the hundred or more slices acquired with a modern volume imager in whole body mode. In the interest of simplification it is essential that predefined clinical protocols optionally extend to the documentation. A flexible report generator is required which allows to compose a page from an arbitrary set of different views of the PET study and corresponding coregistered data from other imaging modalities. The software should provide the possibility to mark one or more findings on any view in a synoptic presentation; corresponding markers should then be calculated automatically for all other views on the report page.

Outlook

The needs of clinical PET have been largely ignored; the recent evolution of PET into routine patient care necessitates change in this respect. Nevertheless, the development of hardware and software should take great care that the research community, which has been the motor in the development and evolution of PET, is not excluded or impaired by new developments. This presents an additional challenge for the software development. On one hand, streamlined protocols with plausibility based safeguards should aide the clinical user to tap the potential of PET without falling prey to grave methodological errors; on the other, the software must be flexible enough to accommodate easily new research protocols, and be compatible with datasets imported from previous scanner generations.

Acknowledgments

The ideas presented in this paper were developed during close collaboration with my colleagues Dr. Lilli Geworski and Dr. Christian Kappeler and in a continuing dialogue with many colleges from the clinical and research community of the University Essen and other institutions.

14

CLINICAL PET: TECHNOLOGICAL ISSUES

Hartwig Newiger

After several years of focussing on research, clinical PET is now becoming a reality. During this pre-congress meeting the application of PET and its clinical potential for cardiology, neurology, and oncology has been discussed. Besides demonstrating its clinical efficacy, PET instrumentation must be easy to use and efficient to operate, in order to become fully accepted for clinical use.

On the scanner side, CTI's development of the block detector in 1985 was a significant breakthrough. For the first time contiguous slices could be acquired simultaneously, covering an axial field of view of >5 cm. No essential movement of the detectors has been mandatory since. The experience with these first volumetric PET systems led to the design of the ECAT EXACT (Figure 1) in 1991. With this new generation of scanners Siemens responded to the need for simultaneous acquisition of more than 15 cm thick transverse volumes of the patient. At the same time the ECAT EXACT addressed the expressed needs of oncology, which were to acquire patient data from head to toe. Such full body scanning was accomplished by the ECAT EXACT's patient bed which enabled single pass whole body surveys to be acquired.

Having achieved this large axial field of view, Siemens also introduced the first true 3D-systems. On these scanners, the interslice septa are retractable to allow the registration of all possible coincidences, even of those between non-adjacent detector rings. The sensitivity gain (factor 3 to 5) can be used for better images, faster studies, lower injected dose, or imaging slower metabolic processes or areas with low levels of tracer uptake.

To make the scanner even more clinically feasible, its size, associated electronics, and environmental requirements have been dramatically reduced. For example, the Siemens ECAT ART consists of only three components (scanner gantry, patient bed, and operator's console), thus enabling it to fit into any standard size room which originally could have been designated for a conventional Nuclear Medicine camera.

A breakthrough in tracer production was the introduction of the selfshielded RDS 112 (Figure 2) with its automated chemistry in 1988. For the first time, a dedicated cyclotron had been designed for clinical use. The approximately 30 installations are positive proof of the success of this kind of approach. Moreover,the design of the system and associated software eliminates the need for a highly sophisticated staff of operators and technicians. The RDS 112 has also proven, that single particle cyclotrons can serve all demands of a PET center, from both a clinical and research standpoint, providing all positron emitters needed in high quantities.

R. Bares and G. Lucignani (eds.) Clinical PET, 131–134.

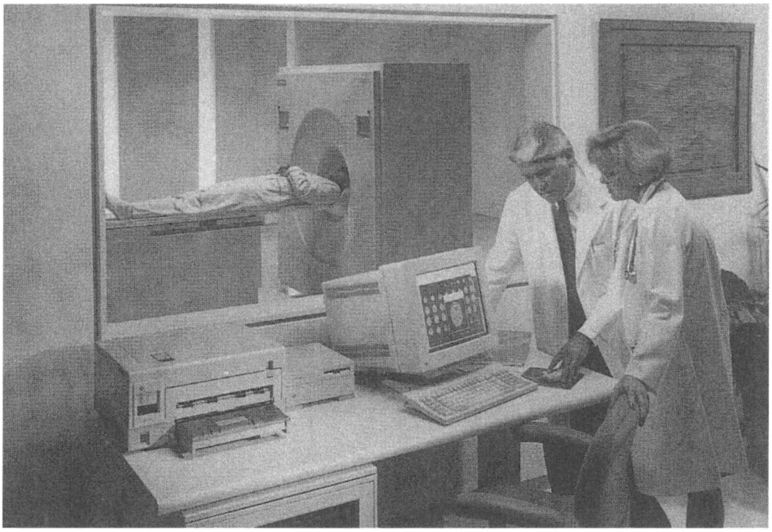

Figure 1. Siemens ECAT EXACT, the first scanner with BGO detectors and more than 15 cm of axial field of view

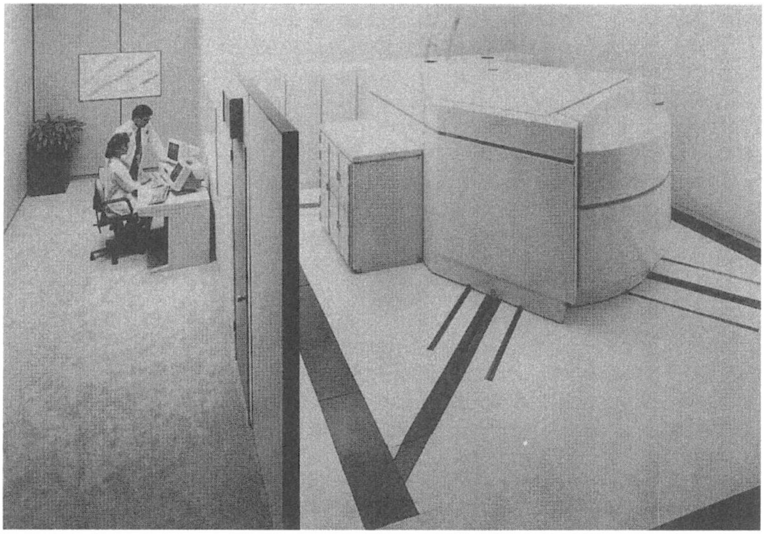

Figure 2. Siemens RDS 112: the dedicated 11 MeV negative ion cyclotron featuring a self-shield

Nevertheless, as PET becomes more clinically oriented, additional issues have to be addressed for the scanners and cyclotrons. In addition to the efforts by institutions like the Institute of Clinical PET (ICP), demonstrating PET's cost-effectiveness, one necessity is to reduce the running costs of a PET center. This can be accomplished by reducing the capital costs and necessary consumables and by increasing the number of patients to be scanned and processed via a more automated, user friendly equipment design. To that end, the ECAT ART is designed to be financially more attractive, without loosing essential performance. This is achieved by using the same detectors as for the ECAT EXACT, employing 3D acquisition and reconstruction, and exploiting slip ring technology to guarantee a full data set.

The new software platform and its improved user interface makes the acquisition of patient data and its processing much easier. Less user interaction is required, as predefined protocols automatically guide the operator. This allows reducing the time needed for setting up acquisition, reconstruction and postprocessing of the data. On the other hand, the needs of research oriented users are not only fully met but enhanced as a site can easily adapt the predefined protocols. Additionally, user-written applications can be linked directly to these protocols. The design of the new reconstruction algorithms makes 3D reconstruction a reality, as reconstruction times are reduced dramatically. The associated normalization, scatter correction, and attenuation correction routines are integrated with the reconstruction algorithm. Still, new schemes can be integrated easily if future developments appear promising.

Potential areas in which further research and improvement are expected to improve patient throughput are for example attenuation correction, multimodality image fusion, and data handling, including archival. Today, the transmission data are acquired most often prior to the injection of the tracer. Also, relatively long acquisition times are needed to guarantee statistically valid data. On the other hand, post-injection transmission scanning requires highly trained personnel. To enhance the quality of the reconstructed data, more sophisticated mathematical schemes will be used in the future. An additional benefit is that this will reduce the necessity for a large, highly qualified trained staff. The more specific a PET tracer is, the more important image coregistration with CT and MR becomes. To link the different data sets, automated image fusion is a necessity. Improved algorithms are reducing the need of user interaction dramatically, allowing fast and precise presentation of fused data. As a result of 3D acquisition and reconstruction, the amount of acquired data is increasing dramatically. Fortunately the available computer power is increasing also. Nevertheless, new archiving and processing schemes have to be defined and implemented to allow fast and easy data handling.

For the production of the positron emitters and the radiochemistry, further improvements are appearing on the horizon. The operation of cyclotrons will become even easier, and the production of the radiotracers will be automated even further. In the future, the user interaction will be reduced to a minimum.

Improved design parameters and reduced investment can help to make PET a clinical tool. Nevertheless, without the clinical advice of the existing PET centers, this goal cannot be achieved. Besides lower priced equipment and easy to use daily operation, standard protocols for the different PET examinations are required. For example, what is the optimal protocol for a diagnosis? When is static imaging sufficient? Which studies need dynamic protocols? What kind of quantitation is required for a given protocol? What precision is needed for the quantitation? What resolution and sensitivity is realistically achievable and needed? What tracers are needed? Are ^{18}F-components sufficient?

Answers to these questions are not only helpful for new clinical sites but also for us as the manufacturer. It helps to design specific tomographs optimizing the clinical performance and the costs of the equipment. Having the perfect instrument and the ideal protocols, the reimbursement of PET studies remains the critical issue. Standardized protocols and national studies like the cost effectiveness study conducted by the ICP will help to further establish PET as a clinically efficacious and proven modality worldwide.

15

NEW DEVELOPMENTS IN PET TECHNOLOGY

Andy Holley

The clinical benefits of PET have been discussed in some detail. However, there are three main hurdles which have to be overcome as PET becomes an accepted part of routine clinical practice.

The equipment needs to be simple to operate. The early generation PET scanners were mainly designed for research use. The software was cumbersome, unreliable and largely depended on the users to develop software for their own specific research programs. This is not acceptable in a clinical practice.

The cost of a PET scan is perceived to be unacceptably high. Both the capital investment and the running costs are higher than for any other diagnostic tool. Health administrators have difficulty in accepting a scan which is 2 to 3 times more expensive than MRI. Across Europe, there is pressure to reduce the overall cost of health care. The payment authorities, be they state or private insurance, are reluctant to take on board an expensive modality which is perceived as adding incremental cost to the overall health care bill.

Easy Connectivity to other modalities is essential. The clinician will often want to see the functional information from PET overlaid on to the anatomic information from other modalities such as MR or CT.

Easy To Use Equipment

GE has made initiatives in a number of areas to address these barriers. Regarding ease of use, one of the most important areas is software. When GE developed the Advance PET scanner, they brought together a software team which included engineers who were experienced professionals in developing easy to use intuitive operator interfaces for medical imaging equipment. The icon based graphical user interface on the GE Advance sets a new standard for ease of use in modern PET scanners.

A typical PET study can generate multiple data files including the patient information, scan data, transmission data and emission data. A complete acquisition protocol often requires several studies using different isotopes. Consequently large amounts of data are being produced. GE pioneered the use of a commercial relational database to help keep track of all this information and to enable clinician to easily search for all studies of a particular type.

R. Bares and G. Lucignani (eds.) Clinical PET, 135–138.

In the field of tracer production it was necessary to have a highly skilled radiochemist dedicated to production of routine compounds such as FDG. The PETtrace FDG MicroLab sets a new standard for reliable automated chemistry. This uses disposable cassettes for easy automated synthesis of FDG. All that is necessary to prepare an FDG synthesis is for a technician to insert a new cassette and to connect the four small glass bottles containing reagents. Of course, it is still necessary for the user to follow this with the usual quality control checks before injection. At some GE PET centres they now have one technician who both makes the FDG and operates the PET scanner.

PET Scanning Needs To Be Less Expensive

A major part of this is the expense of production of short half life isotopes. If you have a cyclotron installed then you have to bear the running cost. This may be unavoidable for a major research centre requiring the full range of isotopes but is likely to be uneconomic for a smaller clinical site. An alternative is to have FDG delivered from a central distribution centre. This is more cost effective as you are effectively sharing the cost of running the cyclotron with other users. A modern cyclotron like the PETtrace can easily produce enough FDG to distribute to 4 or 5 PET scanners.

When looking to reduce the cost per scan it is not just the capital cost of the equipment which needs to be considered. The number of scans which you can perform per day and per mCi of isotope is an equally important part of the equation. Whether you make it yourself, or have it delivered from an external distribution centre, isotope is still expensive and that cost has to be met one way or another. It is therefore important that your PET scanner makes the maximum possible use of each available mCi of isotope. If you are having isotope delivered, you will normally receive enough for several patients in one delivery. In this case it is especially important to work quickly before the isotope for the later patients decays away.

A new 3D volume acquisition mode greatly increases the sensitivity of the PET scanner. A conventional 2D tomographic scanner collects data from a series of contiguous parallel planes which are separated by interplane septa. For volume acquisition these septa are removed and data is collected for all possible planes across the whole 3 dimensional volume. This greatly increases the amount of data collected and the sensitivity of the PET scanner. It also greatly increases the complexity of the reconstruction algorithm. The technique has been available in the research environment for some time, but the unacceptably long reconstruction time has limited the clinical utility. Both the Advance and the Quest PET scanners now include dedicated 3D reconstruction systems enabling fast useable 3D acquisition to be a reality.

Being able to perform the transmission scan after the emission scan greatly reduces the patient handling and speeds up the total process. It is no longer necessary to position the patient for a transmission scan, perform the scan, inject, remove the patient, wait 45 mins. for uptake then reposition the patient. Modern PET scanners can perform an accurate transmission scan after the emission, even in the presence of internal activity. This cuts in half the time during which the patient stays on the bed.

The larger axial field of view of modern scanners, like the Quest, enables a larger part of the body to be covered in one acquisition. This makes patient positioning much less critical and hence easier and faster. The time required for whole body imaging is also significantly reduced.

Connectivity To Other Modalities Is Important

Until recently all manufacturers had their own file format for transferring images. Sometimes these were considered proprietary, so that you could only interface to other equipment from the same manufacturer. All that is changing now. The DICOM committees are defining standard file transfer protocols which are being supported by most of the major manufacturers. Thus a GE Advance is able to import data from any MR scanner of any manufacturer who offers DICOM output. The advent of automated, easy to use, registration algorithms also speeds up the matching of the PET image to the MR image.

Conclusion

There are a number of technical hurdles to the widespread acceptance of PET as a clinical tool, but they are all being overcome. Ease of use is now much better than it used to be. Patient throughput is higher, and hence cost per scan becomes lower. Connectivity is now a standard. I believe that PET has an important future role in the future provision of cost effective health care. By working together, industry and the medical community we can make this a reality.

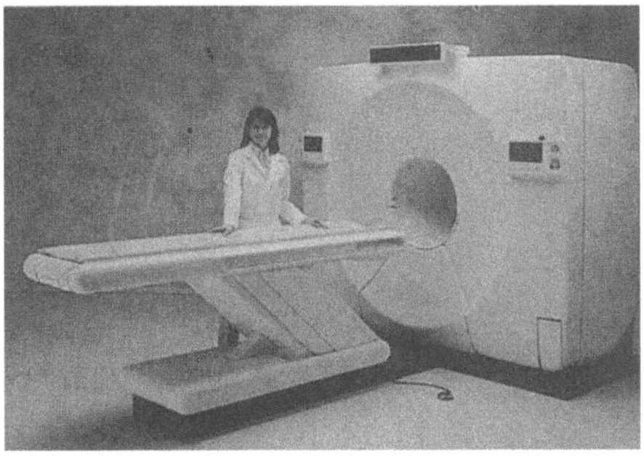

Figure 1. ADVANCE PET imaging system: the gantry tilts to align the imager with the patient.

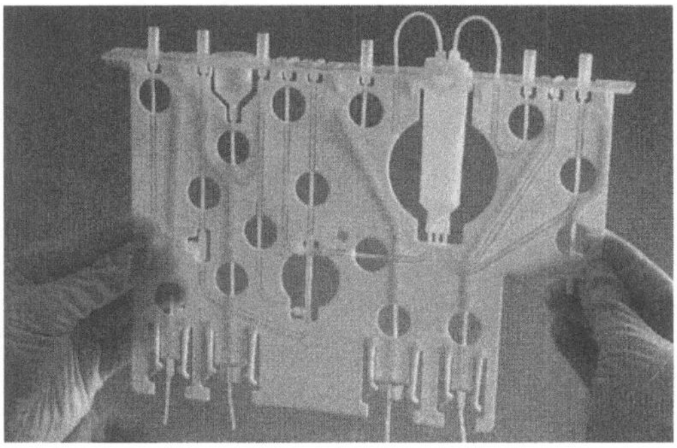

Figure 2. PETtrace FDG MicroLab: produces Fluorodeoxy-glucose in compact, disposable processing cassettes, vials and siringes.

Connectivity To Other Modalities Is Important

Until recently all manufacturers had their own file format for transferring images. Sometimes these were considered proprietary, so that you could only interface to other equipment from the same manufacturer. All that is changing now. The DICOM committees are defining standard file transfer protocols which are being supported by most of the major manufacturers. Thus a GE Advance is able to import data from any MR scanner of any manufacturer who offers DICOM output. The advent of automated, easy to use, registration algorithms also speeds up the matching of the PET image to the MR image.

Conclusion

There are a number of technical hurdles to the widespread acceptance of PET as a clinical tool, but they are all being overcome. Ease of use is now much better than it used to be. Patient throughput is higher, and hence cost per scan becomes lower. Connectivity is now a standard. I believe that PET has an important future role in the future provision of cost effective health care. By working together, industry and the medical community we can make this a reality.

INDEX

Developments in Nuclear Medicine

1. P.H. Cox (ed.): *Cholescintigraphy.* 1981 ISBN 90-247-2524-0
2. P.H. Cox (ed.): *Progress in Radiopharmacology.* Selected Topics. Proceedings of the 3rd European Symposium (Noordwijkerhout, The Netherlands, April 1982). 1982 ISBN 90-247-2768-5
3. M.H. Jonckheer and F. Deconinck (eds.): *X-Ray Fluorescent Scanning of the Thyroid.* 1983 ISBN 0-89838-561-X
4. K. Kristensen and E. Nørbygaard (eds.): *Safety and Efficacy of Radiopharmaceuticals.* 1984 ISBN 0-89838-609-8
5. A. Bossuyt and F. Deconinck: *Amplitude/Phase Patterns in Dynamic Scintigraphic Imaging.* With a Foreword by A. Bertrand Brill. 1984 ISBN 0-89838-641-1
6. M.R. Hardeman and Y. Najean (eds.): *Blood Cells in Nuclear Medicine, Part I.* Cell Kinetics and Bio-distribution. 1984 ISBN 0-89838-653-5
7. G.F. Fueger (ed.): *Blood Cells in Nuclear Medicine, Part II.* Migratory Blood Cells. 1984 ISBN 0-89838-654-3
8. H.J. Biersack and P.H. Cox (eds.): *Radioisotope Studies in Cardiology.* 1985 ISBN 0-89838-733-7
9. P.H. Cox, G. Limouris and M.G. Woldring (eds.): *Progress in Radiopharmacology 1985.* 1985 ISBN 0-89838-745-0
10. P.H. Cox, S.J. Mather, C.B. Sampson and C.R. Lazarus (eds.): *Progress in Radiopharmacy.* 1986 ISBN 0-89838-823-6
11. H. Deckart and P.H. Cox (eds.): *Principles of Radiopharmacology.* 1987 ISBN 0-89838-774-4
12. W.-D. Heiss, G. Pawlik, K. Herholz and K. Wienhard (eds.): *Clinical Efficacy of Positron Emission Tomography.* 1987 ISBN 0-89838-898-8
13. G.B. Gerber, H. Métivier and H. Smith (eds.): *Age-related Factors in Radionuclide Metabolism and Dosimetry.* 1987 ISBN 0-89838-953-4
14. K. Kristensen and E. Nørbygaard (eds.): *Safety and Efficacy of Radiopharmaceuticals 1987.* 1987 ISBN 0-89838-986-0
15. C. Beckers, A. Goffinet and A. Bol (eds.): *Positron Emission Tomography in Clinical Research and Clinical Diagnosis.* Tracer Modelling and Radioreceptors. 1989 ISBN 0-7923-0254-0
16. M. De Schrijver: *Scintigraphy of Inflammation with Nanometer-sized Colloidal Tracers.* 1989 ISBN 0-7923-0272-9
17. Ch. Kessler, M.R. Hardeman, H. Henningsen and J.-N. Petrovici (eds.): *Clinical Application of Radiolabelled Platelets.* 1990 ISBN 0-7923-0729-1
18. H.J. Biersack and P.H. Cox (eds.): *Nuclear Medicine in Gastroenterology.* 1991 ISBN 0-7923-1074-8
19. R.P. Baum, P.H. Cox, G. Hör and G.L. Buraggi (eds.): *Clinical Use of Antibodies.* Tumours, infection, infarction, rejection and in the diagnosis of AIDS. 1991 ISBN 0-7923-1424-7

Developments in Nuclear Medicine

20. J.C. Baron, D. Comar, L. Farde, J.L. Martinot and B. Mazoyer (eds.): *Brain Dopaminergic Systems: Imaging with Positron Tomography.* 1991 ISBN 0-7923-1476-X
21. M.K. Dewanjee: *Radioiodination.* Theory, Practice, and Biomedical Application. 1991 ISBN 0-7923-1491-3
22. P.A. Schubiger and G. Westera (eds.): *Progress in Radiopharmacy.* 1992 ISBN 0-7923-1525-1
23. B.M. Mazoyer, W.D. Heiss and D. Comar (eds.): *PET Studies on Amino Acid Metabolism and Protein Synthesis.* 1993 ISBN 0-7923-2076-X
24. G. Stöcklin and V.W. Pike (eds.): *Radiopharmaceuticals for Positron Emission Tomography.* Methodological Aspects. 1993 ISBN 0-7923-2340-8
25. P.H. Cox and M. Pillay (eds.): *The Clinical Applications of SPET.* 1995 ISBN 0-7923-3187-7
26. D. Comar (ed.): *PET for Drug Development and Evaluation.* 1995 ISBN 0-7923-3716-6
27. R.M. Lambrecht: *Biological Models in Radiopharmaceutical Development.* 1996 ISBN 0-7923-3836-7
28. R. Bares and G. Lucignani (eds.): *Clinical PET.* 1996 ISBN 0-7923-4160-0

Kluwer Academic Publishers - Dordrecht / Boston / London

MIX
Papier aus verantwortungsvollen Quellen
Paper from responsible sources
FSC® C105338

If you have any concerns about our products,
you can contact us on
ProductSafety@springernature.com

In case Publisher is established outside the EU,
the EU authorized representative is:
Springer Nature Customer Service Center GmbH
Europaplatz 3, 69115 Heidelberg, Germany

Printed by Libri Plureos GmbH
in Hamburg, Germany